Elements 4 Optimal Health

The Science, Philosophy, and Art of Health

Volume 1

Dr. Jermaine Ware

DC, CCWP

www.Elements4.me
www.DrJWare.com

Copyright Notice:
2014© HEROH™ Publishing Inc. All rights reserved. No part of this publication may be reproduced or transmitted in any form or by any means, mechanical or electronic, including photocopying and recording or by any information and retrieval system without permission in writing from the publisher.

ISBN-13: 978-1495414909

ISBN-10: 1495414906

Library of Congress Control Number: 2014906870

Legal Notice:
While all attempts have been made to verify information provided in this document, HEROH Publishing does not assume any responsibility for errors, omissions or contrary interpretation of the subject matter herein. While HEROH Publishing considers these tips and suggestions safe, content is made available on an as-is basis with no warrantees expressed or implied. As such, readers use any advice at their own risk. This document is not intended for use as a source of medical advice. The purchaser or reader of this document assumes responsibility for the use of these materials and information. The Author assumes no responsibility or liability whatsoever on the behalf of any purchaser or reader of this material.

DEDICATION

This book is dedicated to my lovely wife
Dr. Tawana K. Ware
Thank you for all your love and support.

ACKNOWLEDGEMENTS

I must thank the following people for their support, encouragement and leadership throughout the years. Be it direct or indirect, I appreciate and applaud your efforts.

- Dr. Nick Fanning
- Dr. Jimmy "Jay" Sheats II
- Dr. Jeff Menzise
- Dr. Adrian Raphael
- Dr. John Bartemus
- Dr. Russell Hulbert
- Dr. Archer Irby
- Dr. Juneau Robbins
- Dr. Marcus Manns (Creating Wellness Centres, Africa)
- Dr. David Jackson (Epic Practice, Epic Pediatrics)
- Dr. Anthony "Tony" Ebel (Epic Pediatrics)
- Dr. James Chestnut (The Wellness Practice)
- Dr. Richard Baxter (The Wellness Practice)
- Dr. Patrick Gentempo (Free Form)
- Dr. Troy Dukowitz (EPOC)
- Dr. Patrick Montgomery (Logan College)
- Dr. Billy DeMoss (Cal-Jam)
- Dr. Matt Hubbard (CORE)
- Dr. Thomas Lamar (Spinal Column Radio)

TABLE OF CONTENTS

Acknowledgments	5
The Science	9
My Journey	11
The Need for Change	16
The Mirror	20
The Overlooked	23
The Counter-Culture	24
Mindset of Stress	27
Get Your Sleep	35
Sleep-Deprived Decisions	37
The Counter-Culture Henchmen	39
Turning the Tide	43
Inside Out	46
The Point of It All	53
The Curve of Life	56
Exercise	61
Nutrition	63
The Dairy Debate	67
The Systems	68

Oils	71
Organic vs. Conventional	72
Non-GMO vs. GMO	73
Chemicals to Avoid	74
Where to Eat	76
When to Eat	78
The Exit	81
Rejuvenation	83
Meditation	86
What About Yoga	89
Try Fasting	92
Mindset	99
Find Forever	102
The Philosophy	105
Controlling The Henchmen	108
Chiropractic	117
The Culture of Fear	124
Nutrition	128
Movement	133
Mindset	134

Rejuvenation	137
The Art	**139**
Press Play	140
MOVE 33	141
Breath of Life	144
Fresh Foods First	147
Creating the Mindset	150
Escape and Rejuvenate	151
References and Resources	154

"You're living in a time of extremism, a time of revolution. A time where there's got to be a change. People in power have misused it and now there has to be a change and a better world has to be built. And the only way it's going to be built is with extreme methods and I for one will join with anyone, don't care what color you are, as long as you want to change this miserable condition that exists on this earth."

~ El Haj Malik Shabazz (Malcolm X), *Oxford Union Debate*

THE SCIENCE

OF HEALTH

MY JOURNEY

In 2003, I had an experience that changed my life forever. My father and my uncle were diagnosed with cancer at nearly the same time. Like most people, to me the word cancer screamed "death sentence." I was young, and I can recall having an internal breakdown. Confused, helpless, fearful and in mental pain I went into a deep state of soul searching.

In the month that followed my father and uncle were heading to surgery to remove cancer cells. Both had surgery and were on their way to claiming the title of "cancer survivor." However, about six months after the surgery my uncle's cancer had reemerged. This time, he went through chemotherapy and radiation. I remember him talking about how bad he felt afterwards and how he had to "flush his system." In those days, I had no clue that chemotherapy was an intense poisoning of your body.

As my uncle's health began to decline, I began to research the human body and what makes it function. Before my uncle transitioned to the spiritual realm, he told me he had discovered that people were being cured of cancer in Cuba. That little piece of information set the wheels in motion for the next phase of my life.

In 2004, before losing my uncle to cancer, I lost another uncle to a heart attack. Finding out why people became ill and how they could stay well became a top priority. It was a weight on my soul to find a better way of living, so I left my career as an educator/coach and studied to become a health care practitioner.

Through my education, research, and experience I have arrived at the conclusion that our health is dependent on a balance between four major elements. Those elements are comprised of Nutrition, Movement, Mindset and Rejuvenation.

The human body is comprised of roughly 75 trillion cells. Dr. Bruce Lipton shares in his book *Biology of Belief*, how each individual is a community of cells that makes up what we see in the mirror. Each cell has a special function, in the community; but all cells must work together in tandem for the overall good of the community (you).

The cells of the human body are capable of living one hundred and twenty healthy productive years of life. Every day we take steps towards attaining one hundred and twenty years of life, or we take steps away and shorten our lives, creating an environment for disease, illness, and early death. Either way, improving or maintaining health is an on-going process.

With the understanding of health as an on-going process, I began seeking an answer to, what makes us healthy?

What is your health quotient?

The four elements for optimal health and healing found in this book are designed for you to obtain a state of optimal health and well-being. These four major elements are broken down into smaller components to formulate what I have defined as your health quotient. Your health quotient can move you forward (clockwise), adding years to your life, or it can move in reverse (counter clockwise).

The *H%* sign you see in the middle of the diagram is symbolic of your health quotient. The arrows depict bi-directional movement, we are living beings and moment-to-moment we are making choices that move us either forwards or backwards in our health. Continuous growth of each element, while maintaining a balance of all four elements is ideal. This is the positive effect on your health quotient, moving you closer to the one hundred and twenty years of life you are capable of living.

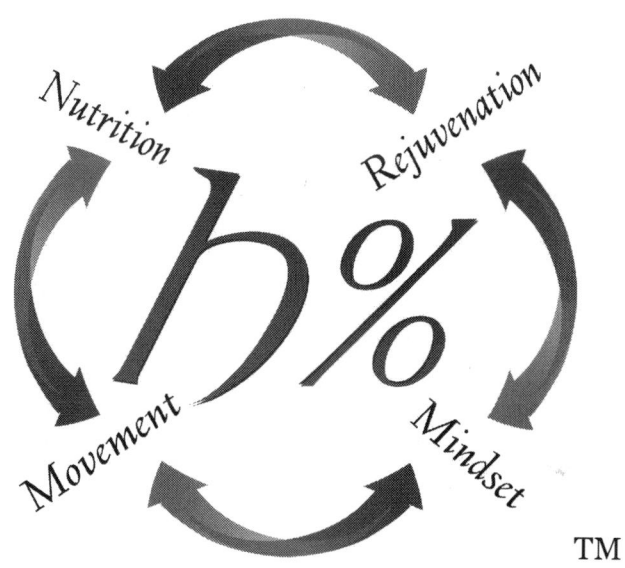

THE NEED FOR CHANGE

The discussion of health in America has a tendency to divert to either the health care crisis or health care costs. There are several reasons for this, but overall the health of those living in the United States of America (USA) is in a miserable condition. Let us begin with the numbers.

According to the Organization for Economic Co-operation and Development (OECD), total health expenditure, as a share of gross domestic product is nearly five percent higher in America than any other industrialized nation. Health care costs are $2,500 more per person than the highest of the other industrialized nations.[1] Research has identified that as a country, America waste $765 billion through unnecessary services, administrative waste, inflated prices, fraud and missed prevention opportunities.[2]

Most poignantly, the missed prevention opportunities are the strain on our system. According to the World Health Organization, America leads industrialized countries with the highest body mass and highest rates of chronic disease.[3] Many of these chronic diseases are due to lifestyle, which means they are preventable.

This is why I consider the "health care debate" to be a waste of time, because it doesn't address any of the underlying circumstances of the health crisis in America. Some take this as an "access to care" issue, which is what the Affordable Health Care Act is all about, but I am more focused on the personal responsibility of the individual and his or her choices. Having insurance is not the same as taking care of your health. It is my understanding that the Affordable Health Care Act is an extension of Medicare:

> "...Services that seek to prevent disease, promote health and prolong and enhance the quality of life or maintain or prevent deterioration of a chronic condition is not medically necessary."
> ~ Medicare Guidelines, Section 2251.3-B

Does this sound as if insurance is concerned with your longevity?

Let us revisit the opening quote. I have taken the liberty of repurposing it:

> "You are living in a time of extreme challenges to your health. A time when a revolution in the way we think, act and live must take place. Pharmaceutical and Biotechnology companies are in power and they have misused it and now there has to be a change and a better world has to be built. And the only way it's going to be built is by returning to a vitalistic, holistic, responsible, way of living. I for one will join with anyone focused on changing this shameful condition we live in!"
> ~ Dr. Jermaine Ware

First, let me clarify a major misnomer. The USA has a system that takes care of people when they are in crisis (i.e., sick) but we call it "health care." We have the best system in the world for taking care of people in crises: broken bones, lacerations, and near death occurrences. What we have is a *sick/crisis care system* masquerading as a *health care system*. Health, as defined by the World Health Organization, is a state of complete physical, mental and social well-being, and not merely the absence of disease or infirmity. This definition makes health a challenge for not only the citizens of the USA but also the so-called health care system.

Our *sick care system* is interwoven with the insurance industry. More specifically, it is governed by insurance companies. Even if you have excellent insurance, most of the decisions about your treatment will not be made based on what is necessary for optimal health. In fact your treatment decisions will be determined by the limitations of your insurance policy.

The insurance industry was originally created to protect people from loss, in the unfortunate event something catastrophic would happen. A good example of the original intent of insurance is homeowners insurance. You cannot utilize homeowners insurance to: paint your house, add new carpet, or replace a refrigerator. On the other hand, if there was a hailstorm that damaged the roof or broke a window, you could utilize your insurance. The same principle applies to auto insurance: you cannot use it for oil changes, new tires, or car washes, all of which are the owner's responsibility. However, if someone hit your vehicle, or a tree fell on it, you could use your insurance. This was the principle health insurance was built on; it is the individual's responsibility to maintain the upkeep of his or her own health. In the event something catastrophic occurs, then insurance is there. However, with the current trend of increasing lifestyle-caused illnesses, it appears the mindset of many Americans is to call the insurance company to replace the carpet in a home in which they rarely vacuumed.

How did Americans get to the point where health, a person's greatest asset, is in limbo for so many? It is because our thoughts and actions have changed, our food has changed, our environment has changed... and few of these changes have been for the better.

THE MIRROR

What about your health, are you happy with it? Do you believe you are in "good health"? Most people are aware that they have some issues that need to be addressed, be it alcohol, attitude, sugar, overeating or other addictions. However, they don't do anything about it because they aren't experiencing strong enough "pain" or other associated symptoms of the behavior. For far too long we as a culture have defined our health status by our symptoms. Unfortunately for many, symptoms equals "sick" and no symptoms equals "not sick." The reality is that neither condition equals "healthy." Try defining your financial situation that way: if the bill collector is at your door you are "poor," while paying bills and keeping him away means you are "not poor." In either case, you are not "wealthy."

This symptom model is based on a definition created by the pharmaceutical industry. Their specialty is finding a pill, potion, or lotion for every ill and ache a person could have. As an alternative, have you ever wondered why you have the ills and aches in the first place? Could it be something of your own doing? In many cases, the answer is yes. We are creating environments that are not beneficial to our health, and we are ignoring the warning signs of these bad environments.

If the smoke alarm in your home wakes you in the middle of the night from a deep sleep, do you remove the battery, or do examine your home for what set the alarm off? Now imagine this scenario happens once a week or once a month, how long will this go on before you decide to look for the cause of what is setting off the smoke alarm?

Symptoms are the smoke alarms of the body, indicating something is out of balance. Do you handle your body's smoke alarm like the one in your home? Removing the batteries to kill the noise (allaying the symptoms with drugs) is a bad idea that can lead to a more serious situation later on. For example, let's say a real fire breaks out in your home and you forgot to put the battery back in the smoke alarm, now what? Based on the media campaigns and pharmaceutical industry advertising, it seems as if most people want to "remove the battery" by reaching for a pill to alleviate the symptom.

THE OVERLOOKED

Fortunately, there are ways to fireproof your home and your health. I would like to share with you my formula for "fireproofing" your health. The fire department of health is the medical system. The primary tools of the medical system are drugs and surgery, similar to the hose and axe of the real fire department.[4] By understanding that the human body is capable of healing itself you can begin the process of fireproofing your health. Your body has "smoke alarms and fire extinguishers" built in, you just have to use them properly by ensuring that the batteries are working and the extinguishers are charged.

THE COUNTER-CULTURE

"Technology, turning the planet into zombies..."
∼ The Roots, "Dear God 2.0"

Have we been set up for failure? Modern day conveniences, while helpful, can also be harmful to our health. All living organisms move, adapt, and experience change; this is the definition of life. Modern day conveniences aim to make life easier, which often translates into less movement and in many cases less critical thinking, as we will explore later. A decrease in movement is a decrease in *life*.

Cars, television, computers and mobile phones discourage us from moving, thinking and interacting with other people. This is actually a global issue; this behavior shortens lives. How many phone numbers can you recall from memory? For most people it's probably less than five, and we wonder why dementia is skyrocketing. How about learning and recalling directions to a location? Or remembering a grocery list? Exercising that part of the brain is key to maintaining its function. The typical day for an employed American can look like:

- Driving to work
- Working at a desk

- Driving home
- Watching television
- Talking on a mobile phone

Based on the body's physiological response to a lack of movement, there is a decrease in blood flow to the brain. The decrease contributes to an increase in incidences of brain fog (a lack in clarity of thought) and conditions such as:[5]

- Lower self-esteem
- Depression
- Stress and anxiety
- Decreased self-confidence

In 2000, researchers from Duke University made the *New York Times* when they published the article *Exercise Has Long Lasting Effects on Depression*, which supported the benefits of movement. The researchers concluded that exercise is better than sertraline (Zoloft) at treating depression[6]. Movement recharges the brain, the more movement, the more charge, and the stronger the neurological connections.

In Dr John J Ratey's book, *Spark*, he explains how "fitness levels" can have a powerful impact on the executive function of the pre-frontal cortex of the brain. Consequently creating a "thinker" as oppose to a "zombie" that goes along with the heard of the masses. The book goes into great depth on the benefits of movement on the brain and brain function.

MINDSET OF STRESS

There are two types of stress we face as humans. Hans Selye defined stress in two categories: Eustress "good stress" and Distress "bad stress." Eustress is the stress that motivates, focuses energy, feels exciting, improves performance and is short term. Distress causes anxiety, feels unpleasant, decreases performance and can be short or long term.[7] Distress is the culprit for many of our health issues as will be our focus. The lack of movement we so often see in our culture plays a major role in our ability to think. Movement, which activates the spine, has a direct influence on the cerebellum. The cerebellum is responsible for the coordination of movement, thoughts, learning, memory, viscera (internal organs), and stress reduction, which impacts emotions.

Increases in stress levels often decrease our ability to make good decisions. The cerebellum functions to recharge the central nervous system by decreasing the influence of the amygdala and hypothalamus while increasing the function of the hippocampus. Very often, the lack of movement causes a decrease in our decision-making ability due to the over-activity of the amygdala (stress and anxiety center of the brain) and decreased ability of the hypothalamus (learning center of the brain).[8] Mental stress comes from a combination of uncertainty and negative emotions. Stress is often defined as the rate of wear and tear on the human body. The cause of this could be worry, exhaustion, anxiety or what I call "negative rewind". Negative rewind is the constant reliving of a bad experience, evoking the same emotional state through a repeated storytelling of the experience.[9]

If these emotions are intense and/or prolonged, it is very likely to result in an assault on your nervous system. Movement helps our body adapt to stress because stress comes in a variety of forms: mental (thoughts), physical (traumas) and chemical (toxins). Avoiding stress would mean you are no longer alive, which means we must adapt to the common stressors of money, work and careers, relationships, junk food, prescription drugs, over-the-counter drugs, daily news, and any negative information that we are not able to have an effect on. Yes, these stressors all fight to be the star on the stage of our lives, but it is we who decide if they ever have the opportunity to enter the theater of our minds.

Hans Selye, MD, studied the effects of stress and classified them into 3 stages:[10]

- Alarm – Classic, "Fight or Flight"
- Resistance – An adaptation or resistance to the stress to find balance.
- Exhaustion – failure of the body to return to balance.

The exhaustion stage is what shifts the body into a state of adaptive physiology. This is when our ability to adapt begins to fail and lifestyle diseases begin to show up, such as digestive disorders, decrease in immune system function, weight gain, toxicity-related disorders, and many more.

A catalyst for adaptive physiology is an increase in cortisol and catecholamines. The diagram displays how the major stressors to the body (toxins, traumas and thoughts) create a subluxation pattern that can lead to adaptive physiology.

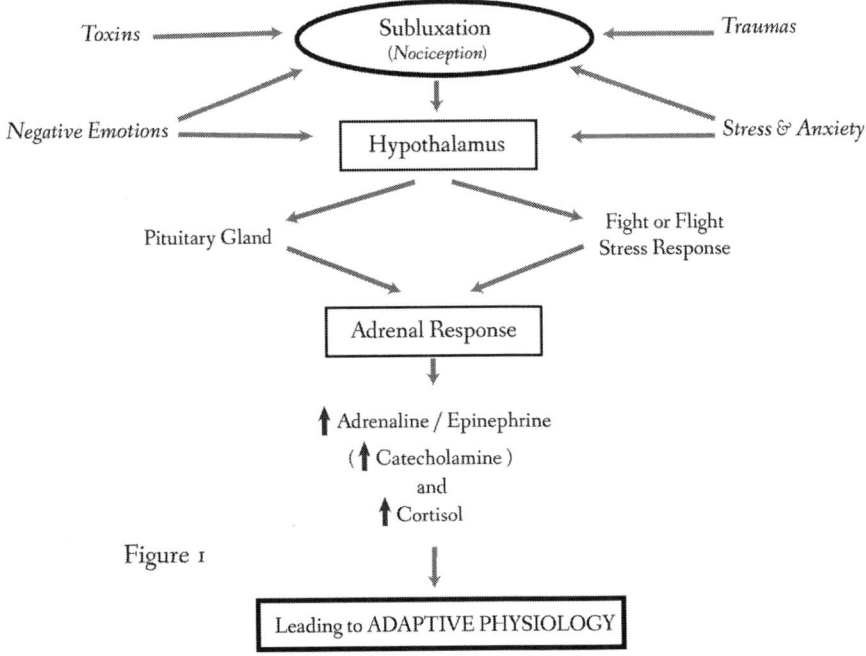

Figure 1

Elevated Cortisol

Increased cortisol levels are a result of the body's inability to adapt to stressors, often due to subluxation patterns. The diagram below depicts how increased cortisol can lead to these common adaptive physiology responses from an over-stressed life.

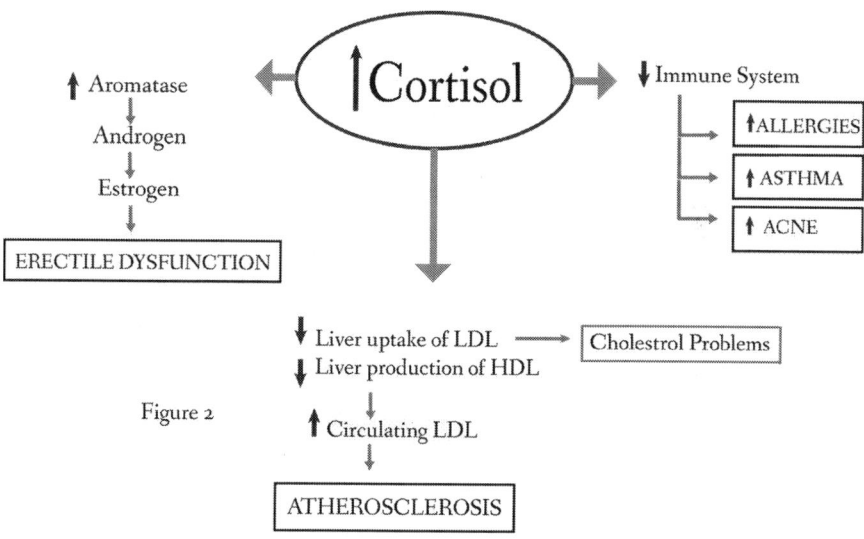

Figure 2

Some of the common symptoms people experience with stress include headaches, fatigue, difficulty sleeping, digestive trouble, allergies, and sinus problems, among others. All are signs that your body has reached an exhausted state on a neurological level from dealing with "bad" stress.

Catecholamine Effect

A stress study performed at Carnegie Mellon University in 1994 unveiled the effects of "bad" stress on our immune system. Researchers sprayed the cold virus into the noses of 400 volunteers and discovered that those with high stress levels were twice as likely to develop a cold.[11] The level of physical stress from EMF (electric and magnetic fields) on the body back in 1994 was nowhere near what it is today. There was no: Wi-Fi, Bluetooth, tablets, smart phones or other technology, which are now part of our everyday life. From an evolutionary perspective, the body would experience an adrenaline rush to save us from being killed by a wild animal. Today, that same adrenaline rush may come via text message, voice mail, phone call or email. The reason this adrenaline is associated with constant contact is that at any moment we could receive some surprising news on the other end of that communication. Of course, we do not consciously consider it the same as a wild animal chasing us; however, neurologically the response is the same.

Perhaps it is time to look at the overstimulation in your life. Maybe your phone could be on vibrate during non-critical times of the day, especially throughout the night. How about turning off email alerts? Figure 3 depicts some of the common adaptive physiological responses to increased catecholamines (i.e., adrenaline).

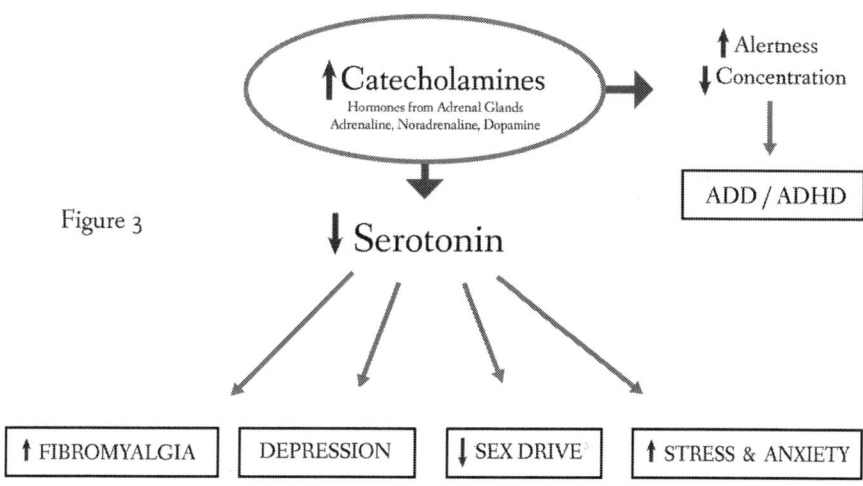

Figure 3

Cortisol Stress Loop

Increased cortisol, the stress hormone, can have a negative affect on the function of insulin. The more cortisol goes up, the more it turns down regular insulin receptors. Down-regulated insulin causes insulin spikes, which tells the body to produce more cortisol. This interplay of poorly regulated hormones is often directly related to diabetes, obesity, and weakened heart conditions. Figure 4 explains the relationship of cortisol and insulin in the "Cortisol Stress Loop."

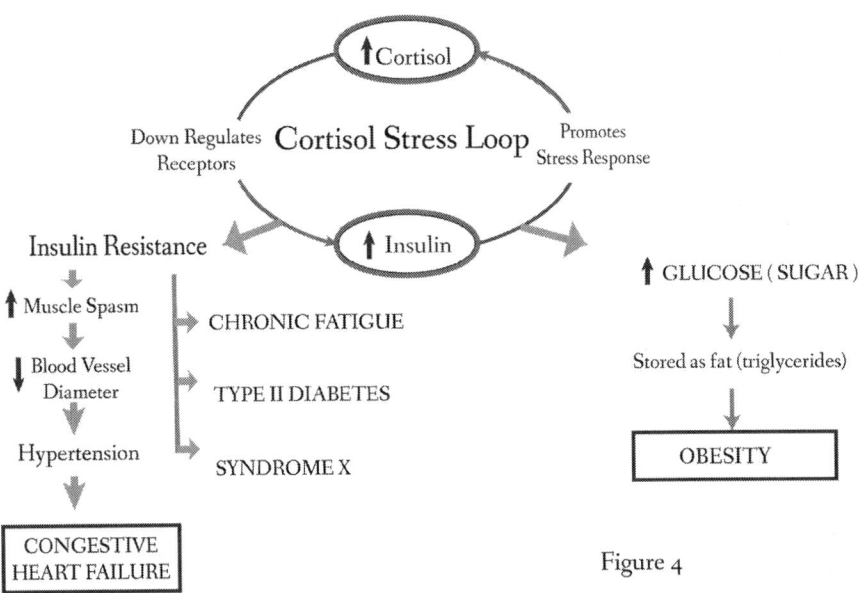

Figure 4

GET YOUR SLEEP

Stress and sleep are two words that don't belong in the same sentence. The signs of a stressed sleeper are easy to spot: the brain won't stop thinking, sleep comes late or erratically, waking in the middle of the night and not getting back to sleep, etc.

Our ability to sleep and sleep well has a major influence on the ability to heal and influences how well we fuel up (eat). Eight hours has long been the standard for sleep, however, not everyone knows why. It is known that the first four hours are utilized for physical recovery, while the second four hours are for mental and emotional recovery. The hours before midnight are the "beauty rest" hours. However, a busy person should be in bed no later than 10 pm.

The hours before and up until roughly 2 am are when the body gets the most physical recovery. Because of this, a person who has challenged the body with physical activity, working muscles, joints, and heart, should have no problem falling asleep. A person who lacks activity may find it difficult to get to sleep. There are multitudes of people who do not get enough activity, and thus have trouble falling asleep. Have you noticed all the sleep aids on the market?

The second half of the eight hours is from 2 am to 6 am; the greatest amount of mental and emotional recovery takes place in these hours. This is also the height of the brain's ability to sort through information and formulate creative resolutions to some of its deepest concerns. If you are a person who wakes at 3 am and just can't get back to sleep, your worry, concern, stress, or anxiety is getting the best of you.

Getting to bed by 10 pm insures that it will be dark out enough to fall asleep. However, some people have conditioned their bodies to require less sleep, and all bodies are a little different. For those with alternative sleeping patterns, getting to bed earlier would be most beneficial. I hear people boast about how they only need five hours of sleep.

SLEEP-DEPRIVED DECISIONS

A lack of good sleep can alter brain chemistry, causing cravings for carbohydrates such as sugar and stimulants such as caffeine. In a study published in *Appetite* Magazine in January of 2012, researchers assessed how sleep affected dietary patterns. They concluded that sticking to a regular sleep schedule, darkening your room and limiting electronics close to your bed is a good line of defense against eating too much or nutrient-poor foods.[12] As Americans we are one of the most stressed, sleep-deprived and restless nations on the planet. It is safe to say America truly "Runs on Dunkin." We crave these foods that pick us up quickly, albeit only momentarily before dropping us back down. Sugar, coffee, energy drinks, etc., have become a way of life for many. The aftermath is the crash. The crash comes in a variety of forms: it could be sleep deprivation, depression, bad mood, foggy brain, lethargy, lack of motivation, etc. The bottom line, you're not moving your body very much after a crash.

In conclusion, poor movement increases stress, which decreases rest. This also translates into an increase in poor eating habits, an open door for obesity. All of these factors contribute to the counter-clockwise cycle, reducing the number of years on our lives by fighting against our nature to grow and develop. There are three primary hindrances to our progress; they come in the forms of toxins, traumas and thoughts, the henchmen of this backwards-moving counter-culture.

THE COUNTER-CULTURE HENCHMEN

Toxins (Chemical Assault on Nervous System)

Toxins include what you put in your body and what you put on your body. For example, fast foods, alcohol, tobacco and drugs/medications contain chemicals that are foreign to the body, and thus can cause long-term harm. Skin is the largest organ of the body, and the first line of defense for foreign invaders. Anything that is put on the skin is absorbed into the skin. This includes make-up, lotions, perfume, cologne, dyes, hair chemicals, cleaners and other chemicals that also can cause harm.

Traumas (Physical Assault on Nervous System)

There are physical traumas that insult the nervous system in one way or another. Two types of traumas exist: macro and micro traumas. Macro traumas would include:

- Auto accidents
- Falls
- Contact and collision sports
- Giving birth (in hospitals)

Typically, there are no surprises with the macro traumas as they are the most obvious forms of trauma to the body.

Micro traumas, on the other hand, are not as well known. Sitting for long periods of time and repetitive motions are the primary micro traumas. Why? The spine has 24 moveable vertebrae and 23 discs between those vertebrae. The space created by your discs allows for movement of the spine and communication between the brain and body via nerve fibers that travel through the spine. Your discs do not have a blood supply and the only way they receive nutrients is through movement. A lack of movement leads to a lack of nutrients that turns into early signs of degenerative disc disease, similar to how a lack of brushing your teeth and consuming large amounts of sugar can cause tooth decay.

Thoughts (Mental/Emotional Assault on Nervous System)

Our thoughts are the most common and strongest henchman of the counter-culture; you already know that we live in a stressful culture. On average, we are exposed daily to a great deal of negative information, which is why I don't recommend watching your late night news. It seems like the purpose of the news is to push something to fear. We can control our thoughts and what we expose ourselves to. When we are given information that does not allow for us to correct a situation or help, that exposure creates a negative stress in our body, be it conscious or subconscious.

Often times we worry ourselves by borrowing stress from the possible problems that might arise in the future, things that are out of our control. Sometimes we even create failing scenarios for situations before we allow ourselves the opportunity to succeed. Are there times you chose not to leap for a new opportunity, telling yourself it probably wouldn't work out? This is classic for people who are afraid to reach their fullest potential. A little piece of advice, you fail every time you don't try.

Cultural Mindset

The true religion of American culture is consumerism; a majority of the population struggles with self-worth because the culture defines self-worth by "stuff." Consumerism sets up the fundamental flaw of this capitalistic culture, looking outside of the self to find happiness. When you begin to appreciate your connection with the Creator and understand that peace is your natural mental state, then you can begin to experience true happiness. Seeking answers outside of yourself can be a long, misguided journey. You are the answer to the questions you have. Spending a great deal of time concerned over what you don't have and what you need to do to have it, versus appreciating who you are and who you can become, are questions that many people have neglected to ask.

"Poor me," is the sentiment of many people, they consider themselves a victim. Is it the choices they have made? The limiting beliefs they hold on to? Is it the fear that is gripping them? What is it that victims hold on to as their justification for being a victim? It is this outlook that shapes beliefs, thoughts and actions, in many cases skewing perceptions of the world.

TURNING THE TIDE

I would guess that you hear more about health-related issues now more than ever. It seems as though once a week there is a new "superfood" that has newfound ultra-nutritional benefits. There is also the boom of wonder supplement drinks, etc. I take all this as sign that a cultural shift is beginning to take place towards better health. However, I believe people are still looking for the "magic bullet." The focus is too narrow, it is not just the way you eat or just the exercise you do, health is multi-layered. I have found that most people focus on at least two of the following areas:[13]

Fitness: Gyms and Personal Trainers

- A $30 million per year industry

Nutrition: Raw Food Groups, Vegetarians, Paleo Groups

- 85% growth in four years reaching $36.4 billion in sales

Rest: Meditation, Yoga

- A $6.5 million industry with an average growth of 7.7% per year

Self-Help: Life Coaching and other modalities to frame thoughts

- In 2009, it was reported that the self-help industry totaled $527 million.

More proof is the use of the words "holistic" and "wellness," in company advertisements and descriptions of services. However, clarification is needed. Let's take a quick look at the word "wellness."

Wellness (*i.e. Optimal Health*) is a state of physical, mental and social well-being.[14] A state where the body is functioning in harmony at one hundred percent and emotionally vacillating between joy and peace. Ingesting a drug or participating in any such behavior that leaves the body's system in a toxic or deficient state, by definition, cannot help achieve wellness. A drug is a toxin to the body that disrupts the body's normal function and harmony. By this measure, drug stores with "wellness programs" are ludicrous. Due to the massive confusion around wellness I use *optimal health* in place of wellness.

Holistic is a way of looking at a person as a complete entity: mind, body, and spirit. This includes the categories of nutrition, body movement, social life, rest, thoughts, and function of the body. I saw a billboard advertisement for a hospital stating that they offer "holistic" care. It's perplexing, as I have yet to see a hospital that wasn't full of specialist for various parts of the body. Hospitals are the "fire department." They have two tools, drugs and surgery. How does chemically altering the body or, even worse, removing body parts, fit into a holistic model?

People are starting to think about their health in different ways. The desire for overall health is obvious, albeit misguided. Turning the tide is about shifting the direction of your health quotient. If you are moving in the counter-clockwise direction, it's time for a shift. Let us begin this shift by ensuring we are able to function at an optimal level.

INSIDE OUT

Without getting too technical, let's look at the benefits of movement. Not just exercise, because exercise is a partial remedy for a lack of movement, we are looking at the overall effect on neurology. Our brain utilizes movement to recharge itself, detoxify, de-stress, and make new connections in the nervous system. A lack of movement, on the other hand, causes stress and strain. The brain receives roughly 300 million bits of information per second; however, we are only able to consciously interpret 50 bits per second.[15]

Positive movement, which recharges the brain, is called proprioception. The lack of movement (i.e., stress signal) to the brain is call nociception. Over 60 percent of the proprioception receptors are found in the spine. This is significant because proprioception is capable of decreasing stress, increasing learning ability, and improving mood.

There is only one profession that specializes in optimizing human performance by addressing the way their body is functioning via the nervous system. That profession is chiropractic, one of the most misunderstood professions in the industrialized world.

Addressing the spine to alleviate illness has been around since the days of Kemet (Ancient Egypt). Present day chiropractic was reborn by Dr. Daniel David Palmer (DD), a magnetic healer who had been studying the spine. While working in his office, DD had a meeting with a man by the name of Harvey Lillard. Mr. Lillard was an African-American who had explained to DD that while working in a cramped space some years back, he heard a pop noise in his back and from that day forward he couldn't interpret sound very well, he was essentially deaf.

There are two version of how this interaction came about so I will give you both. The first version has been passed down through the chiropractic profession and it goes as follows: Once DD became aware of Mr. Lillard's hearing condition, DD asked to check Mr. Lillard's spine. It took DD about thirty minutes to convince him, but after doing so, Mr. Lillard allowed DD to examine his spine in which he found a vertebra displaced. DD proceeded to adjust him, this replaced the vertebra back to its proper position and Mr. Lillard's hearing was restored. This took place on September 18, 1895, a date known as the birth of chiropractic healing.

The second version was passed down through the African-American population via Mr. Lillard's daughter and it goes as follows: DD smacked Mr. Lillard on his back with a book he was holding in response to a funny joke told to DD, which had him laughing hysterically. The smack on the back changed something in Mr. Lillard's perception of sound, and that was when he told DD about his hearing loss. This was followed by the first chiropractic adjustment that restored the hearing of Mr. Lillard. In a sense, the second version seems like the prelude to the first.

After restoring Mr. Lillard's hearing DD believed he had found the cure for deafness, he sent flyers all throughout the country only to discover that no one else had hearing restored, but they did have other ailments that were improving. This was the beginning of the profession. The first school for teaching chiropractic, Palmer College of Chiropractic in Davenport, Iowa, opened a few years later with a handful of students.

"Chiropractic allows more of the Creator to be revealed in the creation."

~ Dr. John Demartini

Chiropractic

In his book *The Chiropractor*, Dr. DD Palmer described the moral and religious duty of the chiropractor:

> "Morally, chiropractors are in duty bound to help humanity physically. Religiously, they are required to render spiritual service toward God, the Universal Intelligence, by relieving mankind of their fetters, adjusting the tension-frame of the nervous system, the physical lines of communication to and from the spirit. By so doing they greatly aid intellectual attainment and progress toward perfection through the untrammeled mental reception of intelligent expressions of individual spirits. By correcting the skeletal frame the spirit is permitted to assume normal control, and produce normal expression."[16]

There are several terms that chiropractors use and that people often ask about. I will provide you with the scientific definition here and an applicable definition a little later in the book. The most commonly used terms in a chiropractic office are as follows:

Chiropractic – means done by hand; chiropractors use both their hands and hand-held instruments.

Subluxation – short for vertebral subluxation complex (VSC). VSC has five components:
- Motion and alignment issues of the spine – Kinesiophathology
- Disturbance of normal nerve function – Neuropathophysiology
- Muscle spasm, weakness – Myopathology
- Inflammation of the tissue – Histopathology
- Loss of global homeostasis (balance) due to the previous four components – Pathophysiology

Not all five components have to be present for a subluxation to be present. The most common are loss of homeostasis and nerve disturbance.

Adjustment – a force applied in a specific line of drive with a specific intent of correcting a subluxation. Sometimes adjustments make a sound that resembles a crack or a pop. The sound is gas leaving the joint space and nutrients filling the space. A sound is not necessary for an adjustment to take place nor does a cracking sound without the application of a specific force mean an adjustment has taken place.

While we are clarifying chiropractic, we should investigate the major differences between conventional medicine (an allopathic approach) and chiropractic (a vitalistic approach). The following chart describes some of the key viewpoints of each model.

	Chiropractic Vitalistic Approach	Medicine Allopathic Approach
Primary focus of the approach to care	Improve your current state of health and function by providing a means for your body to heal itself. This goal is achieved by the removal of nervous system disturbance (subluxation) through chiropractic adjustments.	Improve the state of your symptoms or disease by altering your body chemistry with drugs or removal of organs, tissue or cells from the body. This goal is achieved by using drugs and/or surgery.
Goal of care	Get you to optimal health and well-being by restoring balance.	Decrease the symptoms of your sickness/disease.
Methods of care	In-office partnership, a process for restoring health.	Self-treat with drugs at home.
Desired outcome	Function better with care.	Live without symptoms via drugs.
Rational for the body displaying symptoms	Body's healing capabilities are disturbed. It will take time and repetition to restore function.	Body's chemistry is off and drugs will bring it back in balance.
Perspective of the human body	Body is vitalistic and holistic, one complete interconnected unit.	Body is like a machine with various parts.
Purpose of care	Strengthen the body to adapt to changes in the internal and external environments.	Alter body chemistry to suit the weak environment.
Function of care	Provide care for humans.	Treat diseases as they arise.

THE POINT OF IT ALL

"The function of the nervous system is to perceive the environment and coordinate the behavior of all other cells"
~ Dr. Bruce Lipton, PhD, *Biology of Belief*

Unfortunately, most people only think of chiropractic as back and neck pain. Pain relief is a side effect of your body returning to its natural order. You live life through your nervous system; you see, smell, taste, touch, hear, balance, and coordinate your environments (internal and external), all through your nervous system. Chiropractic focuses on having a proper functioning nervous system via a subluxation free spine. This equates to living a full vibrant life.

What about subluxation? If you are anything like most people, you are probably wondering what the big deal is with subluxations, especially if you have never heard of it. Walking around with a subluxation is like having a nail in two of your car tires. Would you be more comfortable knowing the nails were removed and the tires were good to go, or would you be okay knowing that at any moment you could walk up to your car to find a flat tire or two?

The nail in the tire is like a subluxation. One minute you are fine the next you are in severe pain after, say, carrying a heavy bag down a flight of stairs. The subluxation I am speaking of is the one that causes nervous system interference. The kind that speeds up or slows down your body's natural responses to challenges of the internal and/or external environment. Children and adults that utilize chiropractic have found relief or improvement from a variety of conditions: ear infections, colic, reflux, sensory integration disorders, ADD/ADHD, migraines, asthma, infertility, erectile dysfunction, gastro-intestinal issues, and other neurological disorders.

The medical community defines subluxation very differently. Their use of the word means a break or displacement of a bone, in many cases, caused by trauma.

Remember the fire department analogy? After the dust has settled, you have your insurance money and it's time to put your house back together. Whom do you call? I take it you wouldn't call the fire department to rebuild your home. My guess is you would call a carpenter, someone who had the tools and skills to help rebuild. Think of chiropractors as the carpenters of the body.

Finding the right chiropractor for you may take some time, and like anything, it can be a process. You have specialists in chiropractic as much as you would in any other profession. Chiropractic specialties include family wellness practices, pediatric practices, personal injury, scoliosis/corrective care, some practices also include functional medicine and nutrition. There are other chiropractic offices that mix physical therapy with chiropractic. Unlike medical practices, most of the specialists view their patients from a holistic perspective and none of them are supplying drugs to their patients.

> "Chiropractic care is not aimed at disease because this requires human beings to become ill with a loss of health to the point of illness and this is cruel, expensive, unethical, ineffective and clearly within the allopathic rather than chiropractic paradigm."
> ~ Dr. James Chestnut, *The Wellness Practice*

THE CURVE OF LIFE

Muscle moves bones and nerves move muscle. Massage is great for the muscles, but chiropractic is necessary to find the cause. Let's take a look at a major structural issue such as scoliosis (lateral curves in your spine) or the loss of a cervical curve. Chiropractic is a low risk, non-evasive way to address these structural conditions. When it comes to scoliosis, many people opt for surgery. The fact is, once you get cut there is no coming back. You will forever have a scar, and in many cases you will have side effects that are typically not pleasant, be it loss of motion, random pain, or worse, a second surgery.

In studying the spine and skeletal system, I began piecing together some interesting connections. One of the most critical areas of the spine is the cervical area (neck). From the perspective of function, this is the powerhouse of the spine. The neck is the transition area from the brain to spinal cord. This area should have a curve around 45 degrees, which is ideal. When a curve is less than ideal or even worse, in reverse, a person should expect to begin experiencing a variety of ailments and health issues ranging from multiple sclerosis to migraine headaches.

A trend that I have noticed with several of my clients is the following scenario: Auto accident or major trauma followed by an emergency room visit. X-rays are usually taken, nothing is broken so muscle relaxers are prescribed and that is the end. Two or more years later, there is a frequency in headaches, neck pain, thyroid issues, fibromyalgia pain, etc. because the integrity of the spine has been compromised. Within 72 hours of an auto accident, it is imperative to seek the care of a chiropractor.[17] On the next page you will find three x-rays of an optimal cervical curve to one that is in really bad shape. I have selected a few from my client base.

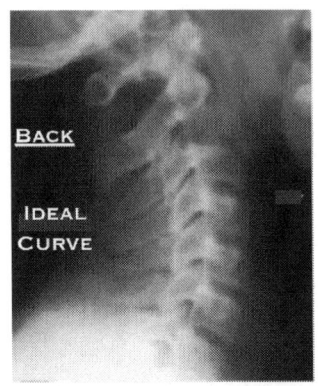

Ideal curve with about a 45 degree angle.

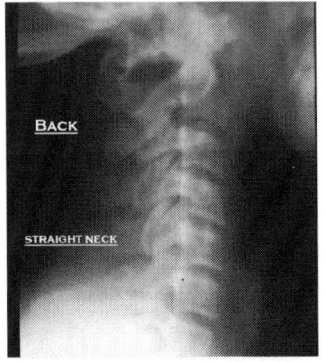

Loss of curve with straight appearance, less than 5 degree angle.

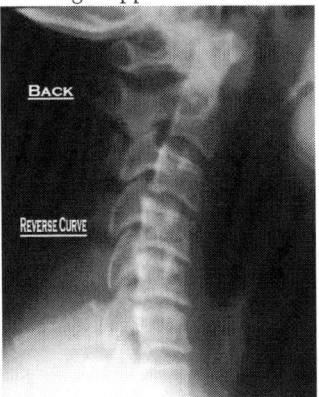

Reverse curve, early onset of spinal degeneration, negative degree angle.

The three images are some of the most common structural changes that I see in my clients. When it comes to having a straight neck or reverse curve, several health issues could be associated with these changes. I have found that several of my clients with a "straight neck" deal with a variety of headaches, sinus trouble and allergies. My clients with a "reverse curve" have been struggling with everything from fibromyalgia to multiple sclerosis.

This is just one example of the type of structural improvements chiropractic can help with. Scoliosis is another, in case you are not familiar with what scoliosis is and how it affects the spine, the picture here depicts one variance of a spine with scoliosis (lateral curves).

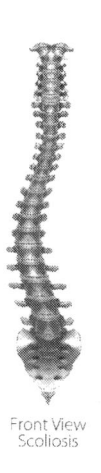

Front View
Scoliosis

In conclusion, chiropractic is the foundation for living life to its full capacity, beginning at the cellular level.

EXERCISE

A lot has been written about exercise and science has discovered flaws in some of the old training theories. The purpose of exercise is to challenge your body by increasing muscle development, heart rate, elimination of toxins via sweating, and stimulation of the lymphatic system.

Some people prefer strength training while others prefer cardio. I am convinced that a combination of both is necessary for exercise. Some of the more popular combination training methods are CrossFit and MovNat. I consider them both to be global training methods that help build strength and cardio while accomplishing the goals of exercising, however, they are not for everyone and should be done in moderation. While they both provide a good workout, our bodies were not intended to withstand that type of intensity on a daily basis. On the other end of intense exercise are slow sustained contractions.

Slow, sustained-contraction movements are not only great for older adults they are beneficial to everyone because they aid in building bone density, strength and balance. I have trained athletes for years and the one thing I can say is that training is based on the outcomes a person desires.

A few tips on exercising: Consider it to be your training time and part of your life. It should be done first thing in the morning on an empty stomach. If you train first, you are putting you and your health first. I believe you will discover that you have more energy, you are more patients with others, and have a desire for healthy food choices. The change in food choices comes from hard training, because your body should not crave high sugar, greasy, or unhealthy food after a strenuous workout. Regardless of your training session, if you are disciplined enough to start your day training, why would you turn around and mess it all up with bad food choices? For those looking to lose weight, this is a great way to start the day.

NUTRITION

Right Today, Wrong Tomorrow

Most people begin their transition to a healthy lifestyle with nutrition. This is understandable; what we put in our mouth is one of the most intimate activities we perform on a routine basis. Nutrient-dense food choices should be a priority for anyone looking to make a change. The only trouble is, not a lot of people know what nutrient-dense foods are. It seems like the more information we have, the more confusing it gets.

What we should eat is one of the most debated topics in health and wellness. There are hundreds, if not thousands, of books written on what to eat. The reason: nutrition experts are still sorting it out, so you will continue to hear about new food benefits for probably the next ten years. I have experimented with most of the nutrition "systems" out today, so I will stick to the bullet points. Thus far, what I have gathered is that no one system of eating is perfect for everyone, but they all have their strong points.

When the eating system is about maintaining a certain pH level, you should know the following: meat, wheat, soda, tobacco and alcohol are the top five acid forming substances we consume. Consumption of these five creates an environment in our body that causes calcium to be released from the bones in to the blood stream to help the body get back to a balanced pH. The human body is extremely intelligent and will do whatever is necessary to save itself.

Inflammation often caused by foods such as: corn, wheat, sugar and tomatoes, produces free radicals in the body. Free radicals increase the rate of aging, cancer and other illness that are proliferated due to oxidative stress. There are several resources that go in-depth on inflammation, if you are interested, you can find a couple in the reference section of this book. I mention inflammation because it plays a role in our health and well-being.

THE DAIRY DEBATE

Pasteurization is the process of heating a food product (mostly liquids) to a very high temperature, effectively killing bacteria, nutrients and denaturing the associated proteins. This means that unless pasteurized products are fortified, with the nutrients that were killed, they would have no health benefits at all. Even with fortification, it is a synthetic substitute for the original nutrients that may not be as beneficial.

Dairy falls into this category. Pasteurized milk is good for building mucus in the body since conventional pasteurized milk has more mucus and puss than nutrients. If you ever have a cold and you want to have even more mucus, consume dairy products. The only common protein found in a majority of cancers is the casein protein, which is found in dairy products.

If you must have milk, the best is raw milk. Raw milk has not been pasteurized, and it contains beneficial vitamins and mineral for the body. However, it is illegal in some states. If you look hard enough you may find it at some farmers markets under the name "pet's milk." The next best would be cultured milk products such as Kefir, yogurt and cottage cheese from grass-fed cows. These have been shown to be beneficial because of the live cultures from the fermentation process. For any dairy product you are going to consume, make sure the milk source is from grass-fed cows that are not treated with hormones or antibiotics.

When I point out some of the misconceptions about dairy many people ask me about calcium and bone strength. This question is the result of excellent marketing by the dairy industry. If everything beneficial was killed in the pasteurizing process, what you end up with is the laboratory replacement of the natural ingredients. Your body knows what to do with complete nutrients found in nature. The fractionated replacement substance created in a lab can have its drawbacks and can also become very expensive urine. The expensive urine is due to the lack of absorption of synthetic vitamins.

America is one of the top consumers of dairy products and the leader in osteoporosis (weak bones), cancer and obesity. In my research I have not found osteoporosis to be such a major health issue in any of the countries in the world that do not consume dairy.[18]

THE SYSTEMS

There are a lot of options regarding systems of eating. The most popular are: vegetarian, vegan, raw vegan and paleo. In my experience, people who follow one of these lifestyle systems have found a resolution to something near and dear to them. For example, a cancer patient takes on a raw vegan system of eating and overcomes cancer and illness. An athlete gets on a paleo system and gains tremendous strength and body mass. The list is endless but all the systems have their benefits, and drawbacks.

Some of the major differences are as follows:[19]

- Vegetarian – no meat, but dairy and soy are okay
- Vegan – no animal products
- Raw Vegan – no animal products, grain and legume sprouts, cooked food. Food cooked at low temperatures (under 118° F/ 48° C), are acceptable.
- Paleo – no grains, no wheat, no legumes, lean meats, veggies

Book after book has been written on these various systems. Most of the books make a strong case for their "system." Without getting into the specifics, I would like to make two points that I think are interesting in regards to food. In the Old Testament of the Bible, people lived nearly a thousand years before the introduction of meat into society, lifespan has decreased ever since; Methuselah (969), Noah (950), Adam (930). The book of Daniel, also in the Bible, is dedicated to teaching people how to prepare meat. A major point of emphasis in reference to meat was not to eat the blood. How did eating rare meat become popular?

This is not a book about what to eat; however, I will provide you with a few tips now and a couple recipes at the end of the book. My tips on what to eat are as follows:

- Wild-caught fish (be careful of fish from the pacific ocean, the radiation from the Fukushima Japan nuclear plant is making its way to the West Coast).
- Farm-raised fish are typically fed soy feed, which decreases the natural omega 3 fatty acids found in fish and raises the omega 6 which are inflammatory, this is not the best source of fish.
- Grass-fed beef or bison – there is a balance of omega fatty acids.
- Free range/cage free chicken and eggs.
- Vegetables – organic and/or local.
- Enjoy all the berries you wish – preferably organic, any vegetable or fruit that you eat the skin of should be organic.

- Eat sweet fruits (banana, pineapple, mango, etc.) sparingly – they can spike your blood sugar.
- Eat fruits and veggies that have seeds – i.e., Watermelon is supposed to have seeds; if it is sterile (seedless), what is it doing to your body?
- Eat food, real food – the kind that grows out of the soil.
- Check food for the "Non-GMO" label – no need to be a part of an experiment.
- Prepare your own food as much as possible – you will appreciate it more.
- Eat seasonal – eat the foods that are local and in season.
- See how long you can go without eating the same foods twice (not including leftovers).
- Drink plenty of clean water (spring water, not tap) – buy filters if you don't have them.

OILS

There are some systems of eating that ask for a person to refrain from consuming oils. For those who do use oils I would like to make a few suggestions. Use oils that smell like the plant or seed they represent. Vegetable oils particularly don't smell like their respective seeds or plants; avoid these.

Oils that come in dark bottles are typically sensitive to light and heat so you should be careful of exposing them to either. Olive oil falls in this category, eating olive oil unheated is best. Cooking with olive oil creates a trans-fat and makes it a food that hurts as opposed to one that heals. Oils with high heat thresholds are best to cook with, they are more stable. Unrefined cold pressed coconut oil, peanut oil, and a few others with high heat tolerances are better for cooking.

ORGANIC versus CONVENTIONAL

Organic foods have been shown to contain more nutrients than conventionally grown foods. They are more expensive but worth every penny. However, there are some nuances that you must be aware of in food labeling. Organic means that the crop the fruit or vegetable came from was not sprayed with the same chemicals as conventional foods. Also, be aware that "all natural" is not the same as organic. Anything that has a source in nature can be considered "all natural." For example, MSG (mono sodium glutamate) comes from soybeans so technically, it is "all natural" and the label will be correct.

Conventional food crops are sprayed with chemicals to kill off the weeds and other unwanted plants. The herbicides and pesticides kill off the nutrient-absorbing capabilities of the undesired weeds. This is in the soil and of course gets on and in the food you are to consume eventually. How do you think this affects your ability to assimilate nutrients? I must also add that it is possible they could come from GMO (genetically modified organism) sources.

NON-GMO versus GMO

Genetically Modified Organisms are commonplace for crops such as soy, wheat and corn. GMO products are from a laboratory; they are the result of DNA splicing and cross breading of plants or a plant and insect DNA. The purpose of GMO products is to grow food products that yield more, resist insect infestation and can be grown in less than favorable conditions. GMO products more often than not are sterile, meaning you cannot take a seed from the end product and reproduce the plant. Have you ever wondered how your body absorbs and uses these GMO products? We do have more fertility issues than ever in our history. How about GMO corn that cause insects stomachs to explode when they eat the plant, what is the presence of this in our food chain doing to us? [20]

CHEMICALS TO AVOID

Sugar is just as addictive to the body as cocaine, because they both lead to dopamine release from the nucleus accumbens. It is a little known fact but according to the book *Sugar Blues* the transcontinental slave trade, the worst holocaust in history, was started by those who knew of the addictive nature of sugar. Most of the people from the continent of Africa ended up in the Caribbean and South America because of the sugar cane fields. Now there have been several attempts to curb the sugar addiction with chemical compounds that mimic sugar. Any artificial sweeteners that are created in a lab should be avoided along with the following flavor enhancers, MSG and aspartame.

MSG – is a flavor enhancer that is also known as an excitotoxin. Excitoxins are chemicals that excite brain neurons to the point of suicide. This is one of the most used enhancers in food products and has a host of code names. You can obtain a list of the names from my website. The reason there are so many names, unless the MSG content is over 90 percent pure MSG then companies are not required to label it as MSG.[20]

Aspartame – found in many food products, namely sugar-free products. Drinking one diet beverage a day is enough to cause DNA damage. Aspartame, as well as MSG, can have harmful effects on the cells of the ovaries.

WHERE TO EAT

Have you ever found yourself eating while driving? What did your food taste like? More than likely you don't know because it was difficult for your body to appreciate it, considering your digestive system was not functioning properly. Eating while driving or eating while watching television are two of the biggest hindrances to our digestive system. These don't allow for proper digestion of food because the sympathetic system is stimulated, the fight or flight system. The part of the nervous system that promotes digestion is the parasympathetic system. This is significant because if your body is responding as if you are fighting to save your life, your blood supply is shifted to your limbs, there is not much left for the internal organs.

Your brain doesn't know the difference between reality and television. Whatever is happening in front of your eyes, the body subconsciously interprets and responds as if it is a part of what you are seeing. This is far from the rest and relaxation state necessary for digestion to be effective.

The best place to consume food is seated at a table, allowing your body and mind to relax. Pleasant conversation is also beneficial in more ways than one. People who have family dinners where the kids get to talk about their day has been researched; the conclusion is that dinner conversation improves a child's ability to communicate when it comes to impromptu speaking, expressing themselves with authority and self-confidence."[22]

WHEN TO EAT

Breakfast, lunch and dinner the three square meals, uncertain as to where this concept came from but apparently, it is here to stay. Breakfast was originally reserved for the wealthy of society and even then it didn't exist for a large part of history. The industrial revolution is when breakfast really settled in with people eating a meal before going to work. In the early 1900s the government started promoting breakfast as the most important meal of the day. Regardless, what we should eat for breakfast and whether breakfast is important are the bigger questions.

Breakfast became popular as the result of an accident. Harvey Kellogg rolled out stale boiled maize, and then baked it to become the world's first corn flake. Breakfast today is still ruled by Kellogg and the products of the company.[12] In other countries of the world, breakfast looks a lot different. In France it is mostly bread and juice, in West Africa it is mostly protein (beans, meat, fruit); The point is that it varies from place to place; in some places breakfast is not even eaten, which leads to the question of its necessity.

My food suggestion for breakfast is to eat protein and vegetables. A high carbohydrate breakfast (pancakes, cereal, toast, etc.) typically makes you hungry and causes your blood sugar to spike and drop. Just like most people, I grew up with oatmeal, waffles, and pancakes, but now I know why I was so hungry at lunchtime.

Whether you yourself find breakfast necessary, there is no question that children need breakfast in the morning. My advice is to prepare for them either fresh fruit, protein (eggs, etc.) or both, as opposed to cereals and fruit juices.

Lunch probably came along with the industrial revolution also. However, I believe the timing of lunch is off. In researching Chinese culture, the world's largest and oldest natural healing culture with over five thousand years of history, I began to experiment with my eating habits based on the Chinese Organ Clock. With this system the small intestine, responsible for sorting the nutrients from your food, is at its height between 1 pm and 3 pm. Eating at this time has been the most beneficial for me, if I only have the opportunity to eat one time for the day. As long as I have my most nutrient dense meal in this time frame, I do not feel hungry the remainder of the day.

Dinner is a meal that I personally can pass on. However, my advice for dinner is to have something easy to digest such as vegetables and fruits, and eat it three to four hours before bedtime.

The digestion process is complex, in an attempt to simplify the process chew well to break down food so the nutrients may be extracted by the stomach with the help of the liver and gall bladder. The small intestine sorts the extracted nutrients and moves the remainder on to the large intestine. The large intestine extracts more nutrients while compiling what will become your stool.

Eating Tip 1: Chew every bite of your food a minimum of 49 times before you swallow.

Eating Tip 2: The one sugar substitute that I would recommend is pure Stevia, this is sweetener that comes from a plant. It is sweeter than most of the artificial sweeteners and I would consider it to be more in alignment with our body since it was not created in a laboratory.

THE EXIT

What goes in must come out. If it doesn't, you have a problem. Let's talk stool for a moment. I know it's not a popular topic, but it is a necessary when talking about overall health. When you defecate it should take you no longer than it does to urinate, if you are eating well. Most people are not, and therefore read their favorite magazine, newspaper or use that time to check email. This should not be a long process, and you should not have to struggle to relieve yourself. Here are some tips to make things easier:

- If you have to push really hard, prop your feet up on a small stool or trash can. This will put you in a better position for your stool to ease out. Investigate the squatty potty website in the references.
- If you are straining only to see a broken up stool, you are experiencing some sort of constipation and should focus on hydrating yourself the rest of the day or night.
- When you look in the toilet, your stool should have a curve or s-shape to it, your intestines are not straight, and neither should your stool be.
- If you are wondering how your eating habits are showing up in the toilet, remember this saying "fresh eating floats, stinking eating

sinks." If you have been consuming a lot of food products or overindulging in meat, your stool will sink to the bottom of the toilet. When you have eaten healthier fibers and good vegetables, your stool typically floats and has a nice s-shape to it.

- Check your toilet before you flush; there is some important information in there. Google the Bristol Stool Chart, it ranges from one to seven, too close to one and you need more liquids. Too close to seven and there is a problem, the goal is to be at a four.

REJUVENATION

Release, Relax, Rebuild

The better you eat, the easier it is for your body to rebuild itself during resting times. Rest is comprised of several components that include resting your mind, body, and spirit.

Rest, if nothing else is having the ability to reset mentally, physically, and spiritually. It is much larger than sleep but we will begin with sleep. Without getting in-depth about sleep cycles, you should know that the recommended eight hours of sleep is not an arbitrary number. The first four hours of sleep is when your body receives the most physical recovery while the second four hours is your mental recovery. There are a few keys to getting great sleep that anyone can do.

- Sleep in a room that is extremely dark – this helps your body fall asleep faster and gets you into a deeper sleep.
- Keep your television out of your room – watching television before you go to bed in the evening is not a good idea because the blue light from televisions or computers stimulates the brain into thinking it is daytime, which makes it more difficult for the body to wind down.
- Be mindful of your last hours – whatever you do before you go to bed is sorted out in your brain while you sleep. For example, if you

are watching the evening news and a majority of the news is "doom and gloom," that becomes a part of what your brain has to sort out while you sleep. What your brain sorts out actually becomes a part of your subconscious.

- Keep your mobile phone away from your head – the electro magnetic frequency of a mobile device is always pushing a signal. This has a negative impact on your cells. It's best not to have your mobile device in the room with you at all.

- Think of everything that you are thankful for before you go to sleep – it has a tendency to make for a more peaceful rest.

MEDITATION

Meditation has become more popular in American culture but can often times be a challenge with all the high demands put on an individual. Studies have shown that people who have meditated for a minimum of two years showed an increase in gyrus (brain folds) which is an indicator for improved memory, decision making and decreases the possibility of dementia and Alzheimer's.

Meditation is an effective way to quiet the mind and hear what needs to be communicated. Meditation is when your spirit is open to receiving the answers to our most troubling questions, our spirit is given direction. There are a few different techniques in meditation ranging from the popular Transcendental Meditation and Focused-Mind meditation, to what I would classify as moving meditation.

Transcendental Meditation (TM), as with other forms of meditation, seeks to aid you in finding inner peace, stress reduction and anxiety reduction if not elimination. TM is different from other forms of meditation in that the purpose is to let your mind wonder. The philosophy is that the mind wants to be in a place of pleasure and it's moving there.

Focused-Mind is where the primary focus is on the breath while you clear your thoughts and allow room to open yourself up to the universe. It has been described as having a nonjudgmental awareness of the present.

Moving Meditation I have found to be very beneficial for me. Moving meditation is incorporating an activity that focuses on breath and motion together. I personally enjoy Kemetic yoga, as I am able to merge meditation and breath control.

Benefits of Meditation:[13]
- Allows for us to objectively analyze ourselves
- Decreases the stress hormone cortisol
- Better controls processing pain and emotions
- Creates body awareness, self-awareness

- Protects your brain from mental disease and increases grey matter
- Lowers risk of depression by lessening anxiety and stress
- Helps you sleep better, improves your ability to quiet your mind

WHAT ABOUT YOGA

Yoga is categorized under rest because I consider it to be a way for your body to detoxify and rejuvenate one of the major systems of the body, the respiratory system. You can only live a few minutes without oxygen, why wouldn't you want your system to be the most efficient? Before I give a brief description of the various types of yoga, I would like to tell you about some of the benefits yoga and the associated deep breathing:[23]

- It helps your body eliminate 65-75% of the body's waste, primarily carbon dioxide

- Massages your internal organs: stomach, small intestine, liver, heart, etc.

- Strengthens the immune system by producing oxygen-rich blood. Also, it is difficult for diseases and parasites to thrive in oxygen-rich environments.

- Improves posture, good posture is necessary to facilitate deep breathing

- Enhances the nervous system; the one system that controls and regulates all the functions of the other systems is enhanced by the rich oxygen.

There are various types of yoga a person could partake in, this is by no means an exhaustive list but I would like to start with my personal favorite.[24]

- Kemetic – ancient Egyptian system of Yoga enlightenment. Kematic yoga utilizes physical movements combined with controlled deep breathing and meditation. It is considered to be a healing and regenerative style of yoga.[25]
- Vinyasa – fluid, movement-intensive yoga that is built on smooth transitions from pose to pose. Often physically demanding, in a good way.
- Restorative – utilizes passive poses, meaning there is very little work on your part, to help your body experience the benefits of the pose without the effort.
- Hatha – often used as a generic term referring to any type of yoga that will leave you feeling relaxed and lengthened.
- Bikram or Hot Yoga – a series of poses performed in an artificially heated room. Perhaps not the most beneficial for relaxation but a good candidate for detoxification.
- Kundalini – focuses on the energy of the Root Chakra. There is a lot of core work and lower spine work involved, perhaps more sitting involved than you would expect.

- Jivamukti – is a style of yoga that can include chanting, scripture reading and music.
- Iyengar – focuses a great deal on alignment, utilizes blocks, props, harnesses and cushions. Could be considered good for therapy.
- Power – combines stretching, strength training and meditative breathing.
- White Lotus – combines breath work and meditation.
- Integral – combines postures, breathing exercises, selfless service, prayer, and self-inquiry.

TRY FASTING

Your body requires rest both mentally and physically. Fasting is an excellent way to help the body detoxify, cleanse and rebuild. Over time, we accumulate toxins in our fat cells. This gradual buildup can cause problems in the future by either mixing with other toxins or overworking the body's natural defenses.

Fasting should not be a foreign concept to anyone that is a part of a major religion of the world. Muslims fast for Ramadan on a yearly basis, Christians know of Jesus fasting for 40 days and nights. Buddhist often fast for 40 days before they are ready to receive the enlightened training. Catholic, Jewish and other belief systems all have a practice of refraining from certain activities during a certain period.

Fasting rids the body of inorganic chemicals (toxins). Fasting is a form of rest because you are allowing your digestive system to rest. On a physiological level the more rest you can provide the stronger your "life force" or "spiritual energy." The energy that was once utilized to sort out the food you have eaten can now be used to purify and cleanse the body.

The four major organs of elimination are: bowels, skin, lungs and kidneys. You may discover abnormalities with one or more of these organs while fasting. For example, you may have pimples or a rash show up on your skin. This could be from the toxins being released from the fat cells in your body.

When I reflect on times of illness, I notice a pattern of intelligent behavior by the body. Our appetite leaves us, ever wonder why? The reason is that our bodies were designed to preserve themselves at all costs. It takes a lot of energy to digest food, especially large meals. It also takes energy to pass liquids through the two million filters of the kidneys. The chemical breakdown of food by the liver and gallbladder is an enormous task, considering they are providing nutrients to the 75 trillion cells that make up the community of your body. Our lungs help purify our blood through oxygen intake, and our skin through sweating.

People suffering want a quick and easy way back to health. The fact is, they have earned the right to suffer with ill health, be it wittingly or unwittingly. The purpose of this book is to eliminate the possibility of unwittingly destroying your future and your children's future. I once read somewhere how the actions of our grandparents can have an effect on our health. This is not all so unfamiliar to you. I am sure you have heard people say type-1 diabetes and twins often skip a generation. We leave biological markers on our children and those are passed on to our children's children. The habits of the mother can potentially span three generations if she has a female child.

You can find the principle of fasting not only in your own life but also amongst other mammals in the wild. Injured animals do not eat because their life force is busy cleaning up the body and fighting infection.

Because eating is an intimate affair, we must understand why our body utilizes so much energy to check and sort through the sometimes-foreign substances to aid in rejuvenating the body. The inside of our bodies are extremely unclean in most cases. Overeating, fast food, processed food, undercooked foods and poor lifestyle choices all contribute to an unclean body.

Fasting sharpens you mind, teaches you patience, gratitude, and gives your body a chance to receive nutrients from food and efficiently process them. Fasting can be uncomfortable at first because we could be releasing a variety of toxins. If this is the case, everything from headaches to skin rashes to extremely smelly bowl movements can occur. The reason: you are breaking down the toxins stored in fat cells, some are easier to eliminate than others. Some of the common side effects include lethargy, headache, irritability and possible skin rash.

How to Fast

There are a variety of ways a person can fast. I would not recommend that your first fast be a 40 day fast. Start small, work your way up the ladder of fasting. Intermittent fasting is a great way to start. Intermittent fasting is when you reduce the number of hours you will eat on a daily basis. You can also do this by fasting every other day or every two days.

For the person on a daily fast, skip breakfast or dinner. After you have been 12 hours without food, your body will begin pulling from the resources that it already has, your fat. My personal recommendation would be to eat your best meal around 2 pm and fast the remainder of the day. This way when 2 am comes around you will be asleep and your body will begin the process while you are sleeping. Drink water until it is time for the next meal between 1-3 pm. If you just have to have something to eat in the morning, try making a smoothie with berries and a healthy fat such as avocado or coconut oil.

Benefits of Fasting

Although there are spiritual benefits to fasting, I will keep this focused on the science of fasting. Fasting down-regulates the brain's insulin signaling and increases insulin sensitivity by the ketogenic process. Some of the physiological benefits include:[26]

- It stimulates growth hormone, especially in men
- Promotes neurological growth in brain tissue
- Puts the brain in a state of repair, also known as maintenance mode
- Promotes autophagy, the act of cells repairing themselves by recycling waste and eliminating and down-regulating wasteful processes
- Helps to maintain muscle mass
- Reduces the negative effects of aging
- Reduces age-related diseases

People who live to be 100 years or longer have a commonality among them, they don't eat a great deal of food. Caloric restriction, which is not the same as fasting, benefits the body in a similar fashion.

Note: intermittent fasting for women should be modified. It is better for women to eat healthy fats (i.e., avocado, coconut, etc.) for breakfast as opposed to skipping breakfast altogether as part of fasting. Women have delicate hormone levels that need to be maintained; multiple days of fasting could upset that balance.[27]

MINDSET

"In the beginning was the Word, and the Word was with God, and the Word was God.[1] [...] The Word became flesh and made his dwelling among us."

~ John 1: 1, 14, *Bible KJV*

> "Your thoughts control your emotions and
> your emotions control your actions"
> ~ Dr. Larry Markson

The words you speak to yourself and others can bring about life or death to ideas, passions, hopes, and dreams. These words can also be the tipping point for success, failure, encouragement, discouragement, joy, or pain in the present or future. The point, *speak kind words.*

On a greater scale, the words you speak are mirrors of the thoughts you think. Your dominant thoughts are what you attract into your life. Have you ever noticed that when you start thinking and talking about a specific car, you start to notice that car everywhere you look? The same rules apply for your health; whatever you desire most for your health, you are capable of attracting into your life. If you want to define yourself by a disease or illness, so be it, you will give that disease or illness life. If you proclaim to be in ultimate health, so shall it be.

Your brain cannot distinguish reality from a dream or vision. If all you think of is "optimal health," what is your body to do but follow suit. The next time you are experiencing symptoms of an illness, do not make any attempts to classify those symptoms in an illness category (i.e., cold, flu, etc.). Speak of it as a minor occurrence and watch how quickly you begin the healing process. For example, you have the symptoms of a cold. Instead of saying you have a cold, consider it to be a stuffy nose in your mind and description to others. It is very rare that I will claim any illness, and my wife can tell you, it is very rare that I am ill. Everyone in my house could have the flu and I would still be in good health.

FIND FOREVER

Our consciousness vacillates between waking, trance, and dream state on a daily basis. During the waking moments we have control, and we can direct our thinking. Dream states allow our subconscious to process information rapidly. Trance states are where learning and behavior changes are optimized. Trance states are often reached via meditation or other methods that take the brain deeper than the conscious state. In order to make true changes in our health, we need to evaluate our belief system and "reprogram" ourselves for the new belief system.[28]

Emotions such as joy, pleasure, or inspiration positively increase the life of the cortex of your brain and its ability to consume information and process. Negative emotions such as pain, anger, fear, worry, anxiety, sadness, or grief all decrease the life force (vitality) of the cortex.[29]

Peace is the foundation for happiness. Peace comes from self-image, which is built from knowledge of the self and inner guidance. This is also in alignment with health: people understanding that they have a divine connection and that those attributes can help them heal.[30] Happiness is a skill that is established though self-image aligned with a divine state of being.

Our culture has trained us to wait for something outside of ourselves to happen so that we can be happy. Houses, cars, spouses, money, these will not bring you happiness. Finding happiness within yourself is the only way to attract all the "things" you thought would bring you happiness. Happiness is when you are between states of peace and joy. Waiting to acquire something outside yourself positions you between the states of pain and pleasure. It is a misconception that "things" give pleasure, which is why they are often the source of emotional pain.

Emotional pain/negative emotions have been considered to be the root of illness and mental dysfunction. Often times emotionally damaged people and overly emotional people have difficulty overcoming destructive behavior. I'm not saying you should not have passion, but consider what it would be like to be in a state of continuous peace. What does peace look like, feel like, act like for you?

Love comes from peace, when you are at peace with a situation you are free to express love. When it comes to relationships, there is no love where the response to the challenges encountered between people is not in peace and joy. If you proclaim to love someone, the response to a disagreement or challenge should be done in a non-emotional manner arriving at a solution that brings joy and peace to all parties involved that makes life better.[31]

> "You are one out of hundreds of thousands of sperm cells to win the race to fertilize the egg. You're a winner and you are here because you have a gift to give the rest of us, please proceed with passion!"
> ~ V.A. Hotep

THE PHILOSOPHY OF HEALTH

> "Be the change you want to see in the world."
> ~ *Gandhi*

Change is the only way to make progress, even though it seems difficult to adjust to change. There is security in routine. However, when it comes to improving your health, your routine must change. This section is dedicated to helping you adjust your routine gradually and sharing a few ideas of alternative routines to produce lasting results.

In order to maintain a healthy lifestyle and fireproof your health you should begin with an increase in "fireproofing" behaviors. Your world, created in your mind, can be whatever you choose. Everyday you have the option to improve your world or make it worse.

I first heard Dr. James Chestnut state that, "every moment of your day you move away from or toward your optimal state of health." The direction of your movement is created by the decisions you make which begin the instant you wake in the morning. The first five minutes of your day is what shapes the rest of your day. Each decision you make moves you one step in either direction. For example, when you awake in the morning, are you thankful to be alive? Are you grateful to have a job to go to? Or do you hit the snooze and complain about how work sucks? It's easy to see which behaviors move you in the positive or negative direction. The key component to remember is that every step in the negative direction is a loss of two steps toward your optimal state of health.

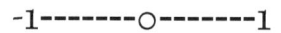

$$-1\text{-------}0\text{-------}1$$

An opportunity loss is factored in for every negative action. Everyday you start at zero and if you start going negative, you must get back to zero before you can get to the positive numbers.

CONTROLLING THE HENCHMEN

Although as a population we have polluted the environment beyond repair, it's not too late to help yourself on a daily basis. You can decrease the number of toxic substances you come in contact with by watching what you put into and on your body. The foods you eat need to be just that, food. Food products, also known as processed foods, are filled with chemicals that are foreign to the body, and toxic to our system. Processed foods are either the stripped down version of real (whole) food or artificially manufactured to taste like real food. They are often the result of food science, full of artificial flavors, preservatives, and other chemicals to mimic real foods.

Eating fresh, local and/or organic Non-GMO (Genetically Modified Organism) vegetables, fruits, and berries are great for your body. They grow out of the earth and are easily recognized by the body because the food is in its natural state.

If you have trouble with certain vegetables or if you need to find a way to get them in your daily routine, start juicing. A juicer is a great investment for anyone looking for better health.

The body is roughly 70 percent water and 30 percent mass. I like to point this out because that is what our eating habits should reflect. Fruits and vegetables are made of mostly water while meats have more density to them. My philosophy is to reflect the earth since we come from the earth. Your eating habits, if they reflect this model of 70 percent vegetables and fruits to 30 percent meats and starches, would provide an individual with a stable nutrient base that should prevent one from becoming obese, or maintaining a level of obesity. With vegetables and fruits comprising 70 percent of your diet, where they come from becomes more important.

Water

The source of your drinking water is also important. A majority of the water supply is polluted with the run off of pharmaceutical drugs and everything else that people pour down the toilet or sink. I know this may come as a shocker, but there is only one waterline that runs into your house. This water line supplies the sinks and toilets with water. The filtration system of most cities water supply is not suitable to extract the millions of chemical compounds found in the water supply before it is recycled and redistributed to homes. Of course the process is a little more complex than I just described, but I want to make sure you understand that our homes have recycled water. However, you need water and lots of it.

> "We will complain about processed food but don't think about the processed water we are drinking".
>
> ~ Daniel Vitalis, *The Water Advocate*

In my opinion, the best water sources are natural springs. Why, because they contain lots of minerals and other beneficial elements that your body can utilize. Since we are from the earth and water eventually becomes our blood, it's important to drink great water. If you don't live by a natural spring look into filtration systems. Most are easy to install and deliver a quality product.

I often am asked about alkaline water and some of the other processed waters. I believe they may benefit people who have certain health challenges such as cancer. However, I do not believe it should be an everyday source of water for people.

Water is one of the life force items necessary for survival and organ function of the human body. The ideal amount of water to drink has been noted as half you body weight in ounces. My advice is to get hydrated first, then follow the ounces rule. You know you are hydrated when you go to the rest room once every hour. Many of the people I work with as a chiropractor are chronically dehydrated, which often shows up as lower back pain and chronic headaches and they never considered the possibility of dehydration.

An easy way to determine if you are hydrated is to take note of how often you urinate. If you are going about once every hour, you are adequately hydrated. You are very likely dehydrated if you can pinch the back of your hand and your skin holds the shape of the pinch.

The Important Stuff

Your liver is one of the primary filters of the body, it you have taken over-the-counter or prescription medications, drank alcohol, eaten fast food or processed foods, your liver could use a little rest and rejuvenation every now and again. The liver has several functions. OSU Wexler Medical lists these functions of the liver:[32]

- Production of bile, which helps carry away waste and break down fats in the small intestine during digestion

- Production of proteins for blood plasma
- Production of cholesterol and special proteins to help carry fats through the body
- Conversion of excess sugar into glycogen for storage
- Regulation of blood levels of amino acids, the building blocks of proteins
- Processing of hemoglobin for use of its iron content (the liver stores iron)
- Conversion of poisonous ammonia to urea (the end product of protein metabolism)
- *Clearing the blood of drugs and other poisonous substances
- Regulating blood clotting
- Resisting infections by producing immune factors and removing bacteria from the bloodstream

Looking at the list of liver functions, I think you would agree that it is probably important to do all that you can to help strengthen your liver on a daily basis. A daily tablespoon of apple cider vinegar is a great start to aiding your liver in improving its performance.

Trauma

"Get Up and Get Out" is one of the most important phrases to remember when it comes to minimizing micro traumas. Get out of your sitting routines and develop new ways of accomplishing your daily tasks. Repetitive motions can reach the point of causing more harm than good. For example, if you are a right-handed dentist or surgeon (or similar profession), when you are not working, utilize your left hand for as many tasks as possible.

You can make this type of change gradually by starting with a daily activity such as eating or brushing your teeth. By doing this you give the muscles and joints a rest. In addition, you are building new neurological pathways in your brain and creating a balance between your left-brain and right-brain.

As for the major traumas, use caution in suspect conditions (i.e., iced over sidewalks, stairs, etc.). Most of the time when some major injury occurs, it is the result of cumulative effects: small falls, stumbles, and awkward lifts.

Perhaps you have never considered it, but children should certainly be check for subluxations (vertebral misalignments). When you consider the cumulative effects of the spills they take while learning to walk and exploring their environment, certainly there is something that may not be right. My daughter finds it entertaining to jump up and land on her rear. This is a perfect formula for developing spinal subluxations, which can lead to other neurological issues in the future such as bedwetting, stomach issues, etc. Good thing she gets checked on a regular basis.

> "If you take a bucket of water from the ocean, is it no longer part of the ocean because it is in the bucket?"
>
> ~ Dr. Wayne Dyer

Thoughts

I know a large number of people who believe in the Creator, regardless of the name: God, Jehovah, Allah, Yahweh, etc. It is apparent that there are many people who believe in a higher power; but their behaviors don't always match this belief.

The Creator that created this entire universe also created you, and you are part of that Creator. So why would you put more faith in man-made drugs over the ability of the Creators creation (the human body)?

Unfortunately, most Americans were raised in the culture that implies something outside of you is necessary for healing inside of you to take place. I grew up with a medicine cabinet in my house. We had a cabinet dedicated to drugs ranging from cough/cold/flu meds to headache/upset stomach meds. Most of us have had years of conditioning so this may be a tough mindset to alter, but it's necessary.

CHIROPRACTIC

"Arm, leg, leg, arm, head this is God body"

~ Jay-Z, "Heaven"

Chiropractic is a complete 180-degree turn from the American culture of drug dependency. The profession is rooted in the principle that your body is capable of healing itself. There's no lotion, potion or pill that can cure all ills. They may provide temporary relief, but there's no money in a cure, so no company is creating one. Chiropractic is different, but different is good, right? The chiropractic difference has no side effects but has health effects. It doesn't poison your body but improves the function of your body. Chiropractors aren't giving you a diagnosis to live with; they are giving you a solution for better health and a better relationship with yourself.

> "The chiropractor restores and maintains the mechanical integrity of the nervous system. Based upon the fact that in order to be healthy every human body needs a good nerve supply to every organ, every gland, every part, and every cell. If there is not good nerve supply, if any part of this body is deprived of proper neurological function, there is no way on God's earth that the body will ever function properly again until somebody restores the flow of life from brain to tissue cells over those nerves. And that can only be done through a specific chiropractic adjustment"
>
> ~ Dr. Reggie Gold, *Valley of the Blind speech*

Chiropractic has nothing to do with religion, it is a true health care profession that focuses on allowing the Creators creation to heal, be fruitful and multiply. Chiropractic on the outside appears overly simple and for most too simple to make sense. However, the human body (the creation) is more complex than anyone would ever imagine. Yet, this complicated structure is a reflection of and often times the blueprint for all that is around you. Everything that is in this world is also within you, success leaves clues and the universe has left many clues within the human body. The changing of the seasons reflects the changes of our lives, rivers flow like blood in our veins and arteries, trees grown like our bodies, leaves reflect our cells as they grow, die, and new life begins.

I began pulling the various connections together when I was a student in chiropractic school. In my studies of the human body, I began to relate the things I understood to the new information that I was exposed to. The human spine has four curves, three that are well known and a fourth, which is rarely talked about. The scientific names for those curves are a kyphotic and lordotic curve. The lordotic curves are found in your cervical and lumbar areas (neck and low back) the kyphotic curves are found in your thoracic and sacrum.

≈ 45° → Neck [Cervical]

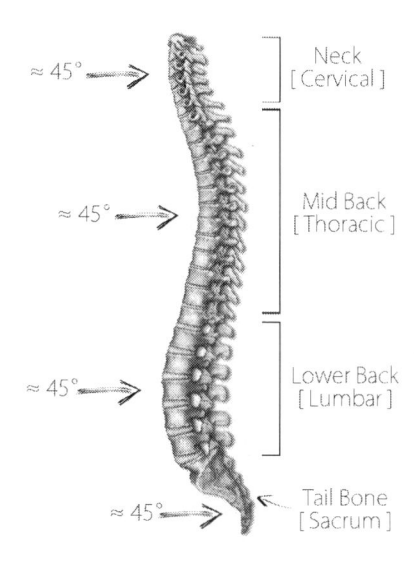

≈ 45° → Mid Back [Thoracic]

≈ 45° → Lower Back [Lumbar]

≈ 45° → Tail Bone [Sacrum]

I consider everything in the universe to be connected. In Biblical terms there was darkness followed by light, nothing followed by everything. Spending time in an anatomy lab examining the human body changes your perspective of the complexity of the human body. I also began looking at various correlations between the human body and the world around us.

There are four major directions that we account for: North, South, East and West. When it comes to the spine, the sacrum mirrors the North, since this area is held in the dark. The thoracic spine mirrors the South, the area that covers the widest span of light. The East reflects the cervical spine and skull, the place of internal wisdom, home of the inner eye. Just as the sun rises to start the day, the cervical spine rises first when you get out of bed. The West is the lumbar spine, a place that has influence of digestive and reproductive organs.

While studying embryology, I learned that the human body begins in the area that is known on humans as the sacrum. The beginning of life starts as a bud and the nervous system grows until it is at a length where it begins the formation of the brain.

The East, the area where the sun rises, reflected in the upper area of the spine beginning at a bone called the sphenoid. The sphenoid sits right behind the eyes; many have often referred to this area as the third eye or seat of the soul.

If you were to look at the curves of the ideal spine, they would add up to 180 degrees, adding the degree from the shoulder to the head gives you another 90 degrees. The degree the feet are from the shin gives us another 90 degrees totaling 360 degrees, the completion of the human body.

There are also 24 moveable vertebrae in the spinal column; we have 24 hours in the day. The spine has 26 vertebrae, which have a right and left side; if you divide the number of vertebrae by the two sides, you have 13, the number of months in the lunar calendar. The eight spinal nerves in the cervical spine, reflects the eight hours of work, play, and rest.

Head to
shoulders
90°

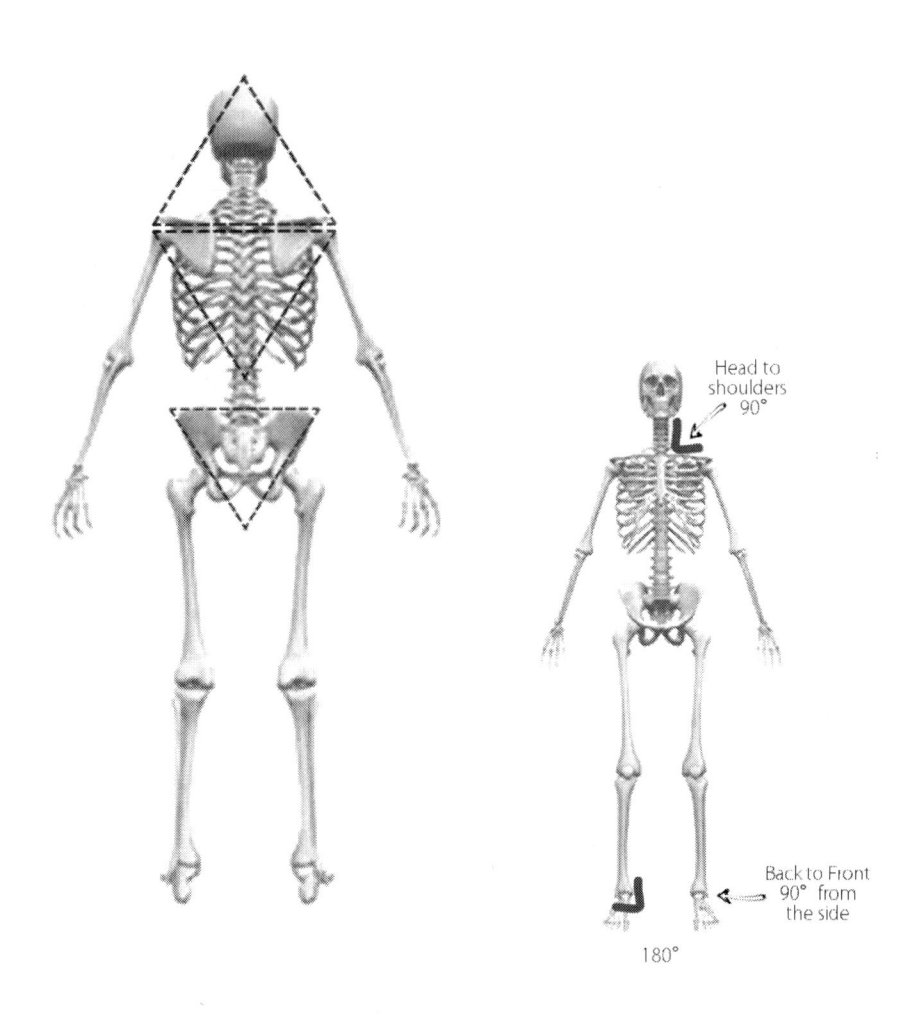

Back to Front
90° from
the side

180°

The triangles on the diagram correlate with the major functions of those areas of the nervous system. The upper and lower triangles represent the parasympathetic area of the spine while the triangle in the middle represents the sympathetic area. Of the twenty-four moveable vertebrae of the spinal column, there are twelve vertebrae dedicated to the sympathetic nervous system and twelve dedicated to the parasympathetic nervous systems. However, there are two additional vertebrae associated with the parasympathetic system (rest and relaxation) when you view the entire spine. I consider this small coincidence one more indication that our natural state of being is one of peace.

Often, however, we are ruled not by peace, but by negative thoughts that impact our health and well-being.

THE CULTURE OF FEAR

Is the following a definition of fear or faith? "Belief that does not rest on logical proof or material evidence."[33] This is the definition that you will find in most dictionaries for fear, however, it could have easily been the definition of faith. Fear and faith are psychologically on opposite ends, however they seem to share a few characteristics. They share: a definition, neither is tangible nor measureable.

Fear can paralyze you and keep you from making logical decisions. Consistent (conscious or unconscious) fear will put you in a reactionary state to anything and everything that happens in your life. In the world of fear you will seldom find logic, planning, execution, or a perspective other than self-preservation. Add a little pressure to fear and you find anger.

In this day and age, you have to be diligent about protecting your mind. We are presented with fear from every angle on a daily basis. It could come from your parents, preachers, teachers or friends. When it comes to fear it's not about who is selling the fear, it's about the person buying it. When you buy into fear, you have made that fear your dominant thought and have taken on the values of someone else. You have also assumed the role of victim to whatever the circumstance may be. Humans have an inherent nature to want to help others and correct a wrong. Watching the evening news about death and tragedy creates a subconscious state of victimhood, because ninety-nine percent of the time there is nothing you could do to change the situation.

What has fear done for you lately? Fear has your neighbor building a bunker in his basement. Fear has parents in every state injecting their children with harmful chemicals in the name of protection. Fear has an entire country giving up the right to privacy in the name of security. If you don't believe there is a campaign to push a fear and victimhood on you, watch a television commercial for an alarm system or a drug.

I'm asking you to take an inventory on your personal "fear meter." Who in your life is filling your mind with fear? What are they letting corrupt their souls? Are these people who sit around and watch horror movies or murder mystery shows? Do these people crave the "unicorn" of bad news on television that only speaks of things dangerous or unfortunate?

Fear has often been referenced as "False Evidence Appearing Real." You attract into your life what you focus on most. Those people who are focused on fear, on the things they do not wish to happen, give that thought more energy, often enough to bring the unwanted desire to life.

Power of Faith

Faith is the "belief that does not rest on logical proof or material evidence," and to have complete trust or confidence in someone or something. What I have experienced in my life are countless numbers of people who proclaim to have faith but are so full of fear that it's illogical to believe they have a smidgen of faith. I was raised to have faith in my Creator and faith in myself. Dick Gregory has a saying, "fear and God can't dwell in the same place!" If I ever feel fear trying to creep into my life, I simply repeat this saying and keep moving.

On Purpose

There is no better time than NOW to start being proactive with our lives and living on purpose. By living on purpose, I mean really setting out to leave a positive mark on the world. We all have talents and skills to introduce to the world. Imagine if Steve Jobs had decided to "play small" as a young man. Would there be smart phones, tablets, iPads, iPods, digital music or my favorite computer, the Mac Book Pro?

Perhaps your gift will at least spark the mind like a great revolutionary such as Steve Jobs, and the world will have you to thank for living your purpose.

NUTRITION

Food is under attack. There is a war for real food and clean water that will continue to grow. A couple major corporations have a patent on seeds that they have genetically modified to either grow in conditions they normally would not, or they have a resistance to certain insects. There are several troubles with these GMOs that have all but taken over the food industry. Without going into what they do to the environment, economy and industry, my question becomes what do GMOs do to the body? Whatever we put into our body is what our body will utilize to rebuild our tissues.

People are into the "what" of eating, because that is where the war is focused. There are religions that see it as a sin to eat unhealthy and to not take care of your body. Respecting the Creator's creation is a simple truth that should be held evident in all religions.

Key Nutrition Rules

Eat food, real food, which comes from the ground and comes from a seed that has not been altered by man. This of course applies to vegetables and fruits, when it comes to meat, find animals that eat their natural diet and are humanely raised.

- Beef – grass fed, free roaming cattle.
- Chicken – Free range, no antibiotic, no hormones, cage free
- Wild Game – deer, bison, turkey, lamb, goat and fish are decent choices. However, I would contest the notion that eating the blood of any of these meats is healthy. I would also recommend slow cooking the meat on a low temperature for several hours.

Other meat options come from scavengers. These are bottom-dwellers in a pond or ocean such as shrimp, catfish, lobster, etc. On land, scavengers include pigs, rats, and other rodents that people choose to eat.

Vegetables and Fruits

Organic over conventional when it counts. Keep in mind that organic is defined as not sprayed with chemicals thirty days prior to harvest. For any fruit or vegetables that you are able to eat the skin, it is a *must* to buy organic. Fruits and veggies that you will most likely not eat the skin such as: oranges, lemons, avocados, pineapple, are not as critical, but the quality of the nutrients might be less.

Most people do not get enough vegetables in their diets so I recommend juicing to replenish the missing nutrients from your diet. Most Americans need 16 or more servings of vegetables a day. You can't eat that much, so juicing is the best alternative. You just may be surprised at how your body wakes up when you give it the essential nutrients it needs from live foods.

Grains & Legumes

There is a great deal of discussion about grains, especially those high in gluten. Regardless of the discussions, there are still some sources of grains that I don't find offensive.

Those include the following:

- Rice (brown, white, red, black, purple)

- Quinoa (yellow and red)
- Millet
- Amaranth
- Kasha (cooked buckwheat)

Our culture has the unfortunate habit of making a substitution when a permanent change is necessary. For example, your best friend is trying to stop eating meat for health reasons, however, they continue to buy "fake meat" to satisfy the meat craving when they should be focusing on a completely different way of looking at food. This requires a change in beliefs, which will sustain the change in behavior.

Dairy

Dairy, in many instances, can be replaced with coconut products. I use coconut oil instead of butter. We eat coconut yogurt vs. dairy. Coconut milk and ice cream are also available. In addition to coconut milk, other substitutes for milk include hemp or almond milk products. Dairy, including butter and cheese, if I were to use it, would come from grass-fed cows not treated with a growth hormone that causes rapid production of milk often leading to infections in cows and increased puss in milk secretions.

I know I just contradicted myself giving you a list of substitutes instead of methods to change the behavior. However, most people will substitute for a while before they can make a permanent change in their lives. The key is to not make the temporary shift permanent.

MOVEMENT

Movement recharges the brain. Over fifty percent of the proprioceptors (good movement signals) of the body are found in the spine. With this understanding, the most beneficial movement is the direct movement of the spine, i.e. chiropractic. I would consider it wise to have your spine assessed at least once a week. This doesn't always mean you will be adjusted, but you should be checked for subluxations.

Exercising should be a part of a daily ritual. Our ancestors participated in labor-intensive activities on a regular basis and so should we. It doesn't always have to be running four or five miles but finding fifteen minutes to get your heart rate up is important. This can range from playing outdoors with your kids, to going on walks, to yoga, to CrossFit or other forms of training. If you don't know where to start, look to the basics: walking, pushups, sit-ups, or other body weight strengthening exercises.

MINDSET

"Peace before everything, God before anything, Love before anything, Real before everything, Home before anyplace..."

~ Yasin Bey, *Priority*

The most important component of developing your mindset is to first remember: you are a divine entity having a human experience. It is your nature to be in a state of peace, expressing love toward others, and loving yourself by being true to yourself.

It is my belief that helping others is the foundation for personal growth. I once heard the saying, "when people stop focusing on serving others, they get caught up in their own [crap]." I can't recall where I heard it but it resonated with me. I can recall from my time as a coach and athlete, when others are depending upon you, your personal issues seem to not matter as much. Which leads me to my next point; there are several avenues for you to lose focus of your purpose, dreams, passions and vision. Reality may seem as if it stinks sometimes, but the only way to change your reality is by improving who you are one moment at a time.

Wake up looking for the beauty that the world has to offer. Trust that most people are good and well-intentioned. It's sad but there are people out there who are afraid of the world. They can tell you about all the bad stuff that has happened to someone somewhere in the world. They believe everyone wants to break in their house, steal their car, scam them, etc. Those who look for beauty in the world, see it. I suppose the "seeing is believing" statement should be "believing is seeing," since what people believe is what they look for and thus what they find.

Developing and growing your mental state is really about being rooted in a belief system that allows you to grow. If you are rooted, then nothing can sway you. This belief/value system is what most people kin to religion. For others it's their spiritual nature. Watch the company you keep, you can only rise to the highest level of the five closest people to you. The greater the exposure to what you desire the faster the growth towards what you desire.

Filter the language you use when speaking to yourself. Often times we criticize ourselves far worse than anyone else would criticize us. One of the words I rarely use is sorry; I don't want to give myself that label. I know you are probably thinking I am extreme, but would you want other people referring to you as "sorry?" If you have done something wrong or wronged someone, you have other phrases: I apologize, pardon me, and please excuse me. Don't label yourself as sorry. The language guard should also be in place when you are addressing little children. The words you speak to them are literally shaping their destiny.

REJUVENATION

Resetting your body is a wonderful way of staying healthy and vibrant. Learn to relax. I know many people think sitting in front of a television to "veg out" is a form of relaxation, but nothing could be further from the truth.

If you have ever watched a child in front of a television, you have witnessed them go into a trance. They are so engrossed in the program because it has their brain over-stimulated to the point they can't comprehend anything else happening around them. So let's call it what it is, a trance and brainwashing session via television. It's not that you are taking a break from thinking, but you are literally opening yourself up to alternative programming.

Watching television before bed and first thing in the morning are terrible for the human spirit. Social media is as well. If you think about it, most people on social media look as if life is fabulous; they only talk about the good stuff that happens in their lives. It's an alternate universe where everyone has a great life, except the person reading the posts. Spending too much time on social media, like watching television, reprograms thinking and does not allow the brain to rest.

To relax, look to fire or water. If you do not have a fireplace in your home, purchase a water feature for your home. Get into a routine of leaving your work day "on the tree out front" before you come in the house. Remember, whatever you don't like, you have the power to change and above all, know that you are of value to the planet.

Get a schedule or routine that includes all the important things that need to be completed. Set reminders on your phone, and commit to living a better life. When the alarm goes off in the morning, get up and get moving. Schedule your down time, schedule your family time, schedule your life so that you can get more done in a day. Living your ideal life begins with living your ideal day.

THE ART OF HEALTH

PRESS PLAY

One of the most difficult obstacles in changing your lifestyle is often the implementation. I have heard nearly every excuse (i.e., rational reasoning) a person could have for not being able to change, which is part of the problem. From my perspective it all starts with making the <u>decision</u> to live a better life. Your power is in the decision, because once you have truly made a decision you have eliminated any possibility of old ways returning.

This section is dedicated to suggestions on making changes. I have provided you with a few ideas of how to begin the change in all four essential elements for living an optimal life.

Move 33

The "33" is an exercise philosophy that I believe can be done by anyone of any age with slight modifications. This is part of the art of getting healthy: using creativity to prevent boredom, which often destroys the consistency that is required for health and healing.

There are several approaches to the 33. Choose from your favorite strengthening exercises: 2 upper body, 2 lower body, and 2 core exercises. The chart gives the basics.

Name	Description	Reps	# Exercises
Air	30 second intervals of work then rest	3 sets	6 exercises
Water	30 reps, 30 sec rest	3 sets	6 exercises
Earth	30 sec movement, 1 direction	3 reps, 3 sets	6 exercises
Fire	90 continuous reps, rest at change	30 sec rest	6 exercises

Air

For 30 seconds you are going as hard and fast as you can. You want to keep great form and walk during your rest time.

Go from one exercise to the next.

Water

This one is straightforward. You will perform 30 reps of an exercise followed by 30 seconds of rest, just keep moving around during your rest. Keep a continuous flow in your exercises.

Earth

Like moving the earth itself, this one is a bit more of a challenge. You are counting thirty seconds (one thousand one, one thousand two, etc.) until you reach thirty. Once you reach thirty, you will begin moving in the opposite direction and counting down from thirty. For example, if you were doing a push-up, on the way down you would count to thirty and on the way up you would count down from thirty to one.

Fire

This is all about constant motion. You will go straight through the exercise with no breaks other than when you switch exercises. This one can give you a real burn, pun intended. This one doesn't have to be the fastest but you need to push to complete the reps without stopping.

The objective of the exercises is to get your heart rate up and your blood pumping. Yes, even the Earth exercises will get you to break a sweat. Done properly, these are some great workouts for the beginner, those short on time, and those who can't afford a gym membership. The speed and/or duration of the exercises adds a level of cardio to the routine. These routines challenge you to the point of a short cardio workout. You can also add a short run to your routine every now and again.

Optional Equipment:
- Exercise ball
- Resistance bands
- Dumb bells

Sample Routines:
Routine 1
- Pushups
- Air squats
- Crunches
- Burpee/Squat thrust
- Supermans
- Planks

Routine 2
- Squat to overhead Press, with resistance band
- One-arm row, with resistance band
- Band boxing, with resistance band
- Lunges
- Donkey kicks
- Side planks

BREATH OF LIFE

Nearly all disease is associated with the lack of toxins being removed from the body. The three major methods of toxin removal include the digestive system, lymphatic system and respiratory system. When it comes to breathing, I have found that most people have forgotten how to breathe effectively. When we were infants we had it, as we matured, we lost it.

My introduction to the importance of breathing came when I was coaching track and field. I studied breathing patterns to help aid my athletes in competition as well as recovery. I later transitioned this study to the health benefits of breathing, other than staying alive. Deep abdominal breathing, what we all did as infants, is extremely beneficial considering it helps: expel carbon dioxide from the body, oxygenate the tissues of the body and bring about an overall feeling of relaxation.

Take a moment and pay attention to the number of times you breathe in a one-minute interval. I have observed that most people who have a difficult time relaxing breathe eighteen or more times per minute. This is common for shallow breathers and those people who are easily alarmed. It is difficult for a person to be relaxed while breathing so rapidly.

Relax

Every breath you take that is less than 18 breaths in a minute calms your nervous system and brings you closer to your Creator by distancing you farther from your worldly concerns. There are two reasons, when you slow down your breath you calm your body and your mind begins to focus on staying alive. You reconnect the body and the mind, because despite your own doing, your body's primary objective is to stay alive at all cost. So when upset over something in life, take long and slow breaths until you regain focus to the bigger picture, regardless of what your brain says. Slowing your breath to three or less breaths per minute is the ultimate goal in aligning your mind, body and soul with the Creator.

Breathing Exercises

For beginners, start with the number three. Sit-up straight or stand, take note of your stomach area. Your goal is to make your stomach balloon out while you breathe in and you want your belly button touch your spine, when you breathe out (in theory). Breathe in while counting to five, hold it for five and blow it out holding it for five. Make 10 to 20 deep breaths part of your daily routine. If you can, get outdoors to do it. Spend at least five minutes if not ten, reconnecting with yourself on a daily basis. Do this as often as you would like.

Beginners: Breathe in for a count of four, in your head count "one thousand one, one thousand two," up to four. Once you have filled up your abdomen, hold it for another four-second count and then blow the breath out while counting to four in your head. This a daily exercise that you can perform at any time. Once you have mastered this level, take it to a five count.

FRESH FOODS FIRST

Dr. James Chestnut first introduced me to the idea of fresh fiber first. I found this to be an effective method of transitioning a person to eating healthier. Unfortunately, fresh fiber such as raw vegetables, berries and leafy greens are new to some people. If you are a person who struggles with eating vegetables, I recommend juicing.

There will be several recipes on my website but I wanted to share a few with you. For my juices I like to use celery and cucumber as a base. Cucumber and Celery have several health benefits including:

- Healing of diseased gums
- Stabilizing blood pressure
- Help flush toxins
- Fight muscle and joint pain
- Help lower cholesterol
- Potential to cure digestive disorders
- Cancer fighting abilities

For this drink, I use a juicer. I start with the kale, since it's the most difficult to juice. Follow with celery, lemon and apple, in that order.

The Cleaner:
- 1 green Apple
- 4 Leaves of kale
- 4 Stalks of Celery
- 1 Cucumber
- 1 small lemon

After a tough workout, you have effectively increased the level of free radicals in your body. *The Recovery* is intended to super charge your antioxidant levels while aiding in the healing/recovery process.

The Recovery:
- 2 Frozen Bananas
- 1 ½ tbsp. Raw Cacao powder
- 1 cup hemp milk (add more for less consistency)
- ¼ cup frozen blue berries
- 1 tbsp. Acai Powder
- 1 tbsp. Cod-liver oil

Blend in Vitamix and enjoy

I live by the 70/30 model I spoke of earlier in the book. So I would like to share with you one of my meat dishes. Meat that is cooked slowly has its advantages. Slow cooked meats are tender, they do not have to be browned and they are often easier to digest. The following is one of my many recipes for free-range chicken. This is prepared by using a slow cooker.

- Whole Organic Free-Range Chicken
- 1 handful of Cilantro
- 3 cloves of fresh garlic
- 2 tbsp minced garlic
- ½ white or yellow onion
- Lemon Pepper seasoning
- Lemon juice

Wash the chicken, and remove the inside pouch. Stuff the inside of the chicken with cilantro (a handful), onion, and the fresh garlic (smash the garlic). Place the entire chicken in the slow cooker. Rub lightly with coconut oil, minced garlic and lemon pepper. Cut two quarters of the lemon and place directly on the chicken, take the other half and squeeze the lemon juice over the rest of the chicken when finished. Cook on low for four to six hours in the slow cooker and enjoy!

CREATING THE MINDSET

Affirmations and Questions

Affirmations are self-declarations of your truth. While beneficial to state aloud and daily, they will vary from person to person. I know people who have affirmations that are a few paragraphs and others that are a few sentences. The purpose of an affirmation is to help you fuel your life vision and/or to focus your energy on productive behaviors.

Questions are a powerful tool that you can utilize to stimulate your creativity. Asking yourself the hard questions, forces your brain to seek an answer. Asking yourself questions like: "how long it will take me to get my health to where I want it?" "What would I need to do be able to afford xyz?" These are examples of questions you could ask yourself before you go to bed at night. Give yourself a day or two and see what ideas manifest.

ESCAPE AND REJUVENATE

The ability to rebuild is critical to your survival. There are times when you need to step away from your daily activities to refresh your mind, body, and soul. If you are thinking about vacation, shake it off. Let's look at something we can do on a daily basis that will help us detach from our reality and come back a little fresher.

Here are my suggestions for detaching from your reality:

- Before you tell a story about something "bad" that happened in your day you must be able to communicate how you grew from the situation. This could be what you learned about yourself, what you learned about another person, what you gained from the experience, or a more effective way this could have been presented.
- Take the television and all electronic devices out of your bedroom. I know, you use your cell phone for an alarm clock, right? Well put it in another room, even if it's the bathroom just take it out of your room and place it face down on the counter.
- End all communications with outside people at least two hours before bedtime, no need to be processing someone's issues while you rest and resolve your own.

- Write down everything you were grateful for that day. Follow that with the questions to which you desire answers.

When it is all said and done, I am a wellness practitioner that is in the relationship business. My goal is for you to have the best relationship you can have with yourself so that you may be able to be at your best with your family, friends, children, and people of the world. *Elements4.me* is an extension of this text and has been created in the spirit of sharing information, challenging you to be your best and supporting you with a community of people who have similar goals.

Reclaiming your health is an act of love, a show of affection for oneself. My mission is to work with people who truly love themselves and desire to take their self-love even higher. My definition of someone who loves him or herself includes people who do not do things to harm themselves physically, mentally or spiritually. Life is a blessing, and every day I thank the Creator for giving me another day. It is my hope that this book, at a minimum, will allow you to discover ways to upgrade your life.

"If children were raised with a better understanding of the human body as an amazing and divinely-created vehicle, how it functions, how it is healed and harmed, they would be more likely to take care of, enhance and protect it."

~ Jeff Menzise, PhD, *Dumbin' Down*

"....they want to know what the end game is, this is the end game. Everybody here with a camera, everybody here with a smart phone, everyone here with a voice, do your job and spread the word. Make it grow, it's about growth now, we have to grow, and that's the point! I love ya'll!"

~ Talib Kweli, *Prisoner of Conscious*

REFERENCES & RESOURCES

1. Dr. J. Mercola. *The True Cost of a Flawed Healthcare Paradigm.* <mercola.com>.
2. "National Prevention Strategy: America's Plan for Better Health and Wellness." *Centers for Disease Control and Prevention.* Centers for Disease Control and Prevention, 17 Jan. 2014.
3. "Obesity." WHO, Global Health Observatory. <www.who.int/gho/ncd/risk_factors/obesity_text/en/>.
4. Chestnut, Dr. James. "Scientific and Philosophical Validation of the Chiropractic Wellness Paradigm." Mar. 2008. Lecture.
5. Hobbs, Christopher. Stress & natural healing. Santa Cruz, CA: Botanica P, 1997
6. "Duke Today." *Exercise has long-lasting effect on depression.* Duke Today. 22 Sep. 2000 <https://today.duke.edu/2000/09/exercise922.html>.
7. "Types of Stressors (Eustress vs. Distress)." - Dealing with Stress and Anxiety Management – Coping Mechanisms from MentalHelp.net. 30 Jun. 2008 <http://www.mentalhelp.net/poc/view_doc.php?type=doc&id=15644>.
8. Hobbs, Christopher. Stress & natural healing. Santa Cruz, CA: Botanica P, 1997.
9. Ra Un Nefer Amen, 2011. *Metu Netur Vol 5: Keys to Health and Longevity.*

10. "Hans Selye's General Adaptation Syndrome." Classic stages of chronic stress. 08 Mar. 2014 <http://www.essenceofstressrelief.com/general-adaptation-syndrome.html>.

11. Sheldon Cohen. "Psychological Stress, Immunity, and Upper Respiratory Infections," *Current Directions in Psychological Science*, June 1996. 5, 3. 86-89.

12. "How lack of sleep affects the brain and may increase appetite, weight gain." Scope Blog RSS. 13 Mar. 2014 <http://scopeblog.stanford.edu/2012/01/18/how-lack-of-sleep-affects-the-brain-and-may-increase-appetite-weight-gain/>.

13. "Gym, Health & Fitness Clubs in the US: Market Research Report." *Gym, Health & Fitness Clubs in the US Market Research*. Feb. 2014.

14. Chestnut, James L. The 14 foundational premises for the scientific and philosophical validation of the chiropractic wellness paradigm. Victoria, B.C.: Wellness Practice, 2003.

15. Chestnut, James L. The 14 foundational premises for the scientific and philosophical validation of the chiropractic wellness paradigm. Victoria, B.C.: Wellness Practice, 2003.

16. Palmer, D.D. The Chiropractor. Portland, OR: Portland Printing House Company, 1914.

17. Murphy, Dr Dan. "Posture Neurology and Health." Atlanta. Nov. 2010.

18. "Facts and Statistics." *International Osteoporosis Foundation*. <www.iofbonehealth.org/facts-statistics#category-28Foundation>.

19. Lipton, Bruce H. The biology of belief. Memphis, TN: Spirit 2000, Inc., 2003.

20. Mercola, Dr. "Eating This Could Turn Your Gut into a Living Pesticide Factory." <u>Mercola.com</u>. May-June 2012. <http://articles.mercola.com/sites/articles/archive/2012/05/29/genetically-modified-crops-insects-emerged.aspx>.
21. "What Foods To Avoid?" <u>What Foods Should I Avoid?</u> 13 Mar. 2013 <http://www.msgtruth.org/avoid.htm>.
22. "Building Self-Esteem in Your Kids." Shana Schutte. <www.focusonthefamily.com>.
23. "Benefits of Yoga." <dailyburn.com/life/fitness/health-benefits-yoga/>.
24. Kemetic Yoga. <kemeticyoga.com>.
25. Ratey, John J., and Eric Hagerman. <u>Spark: The revolutionary new science of exercise and the brain</u>. New York: Little, Brown, 2008.
26. "10 Incredible Health Benefits of Fasting." Dr. Biodun Awosusi. <voices.yahoo.com/10-incredible-health-benefits-fasting-11621130.html>.
27. Virgin, JJ. Interview. Audio blog post. <u>Bulletproofexec.com</u>. <Bulletproofexec.com>
28. Ra Un Nefer Amen, 2011. *Metu Netur Vol 5: Keys to Health and Longevity.*
29. Ra Un Nefer Amen, 2011. *Metu Netur Vol 5: Keys to Health and Longevity.*
30. Ra Un Nefer Amen, 2011. *Metu Netur Vol 5: Keys to Health and Longevity.*
31. Ra Un Nefer Amen, 2011. *Metu Netur Vol 5: Keys to Health and Longevity.*

32. "Liver, Biliary, and Pancreatic Disorders." <u>Liver, Biliary, and Pancreatic Disorders</u>. 16 Mar. 2014 <http://medicalcenter.osu.edu/patientcare/healthcare_services/liver_biliary_pancreatic_disease/Pages/index.aspx>.
33. "Faith." *Wikipedia*. Wikimedia Foundation, 03 Sept. 2013.
34. Chestnut, James L. <u>The 14 foundational premises for the scientific and philosophical validation of the chiropractic wellness paradigm</u>. Victoria, B.C.: Wellness Practice, 2003.

Diagrams:

- Figure 1 – James L Chestnut DC, CCWP. "The Innate State of Mind & Emotional Hygiene," Extrapolated from the *Neurology of Negative Mind and Body Thoughts and Adaptation & Illness and Positive Mind and Body Thought and Homeostasis & Health* Victoria, B.C.: Wellness Practice, 2005.
- Figures 2, 3, 4 – Adrian Raphael DC, CCWP. Extrapolated from the *Adaptive Physiology to Chronic Stress: A Common Denominator in Lifestyle Disease*.

Other Resources for Health Information

Podcasts:
- The Model Health Show – Shawn Stevenson
- Underground Wellness Radio – Sean Croxton
- Bulletproof Executive Radio – Dave Asprey

Websites:
- DrFabMancini.com
- TheShawnStevensonModel.com
- Undergroundwellness.com
- SpinalColumnRadio.com
- Fitlife.tv
- KoyaWebb.com
- AshleyTurner.org
- Well.org
- Mindonthematter.com
- Mercola.com
- GreenMedinfo.com
- Foodmatters.tv
- PreventDisease.com
- Icpa4kids.org
- KatieFell.com
- Squattypotty.com/?Click=46067

Supplements:
For the following: email *code@heroh.com* for discount and/or purchase code information.
- *Innatechoice.com* – supplements
- *Emersonecologics.com* – supplements
- *Perfectsupplements.com* – super food supplements
- *Sunfoods.com* – super food supplements
- *UpgradedSelf.com* – super food supplements
- *IntelliSkin.net* – clothing, posture improvement

Books:
- *Spark* – John J Ratey, MD
- *Wheat Belly* – William Davis, MD
- *Anti-Inflammatory Diet* – Jennifer Sather
- *Take Control of Your Health* – Joseph Mercola, DO
- *Health and Nutrition Secrets* – Russell Blaylock, MD
- *Excitotoxins* – Russell Blaylock, MD

www.Elements4.me

www.DrJWare.com

Made in the USA
Lexington, KY
27 February 2018